/1450

Clinical Reactions to Food

Clinical Reactions to Food

Edited by

M. H. Lessof
Professor of Medicine
Guy's Hospital Medical School
London

A Wiley Medical Publication

JOHN WILEY & SONS

Chichester · New York · Brisbane · Toronto · Singapore

Library of Congress Cataloging in Publication Data:

Main entry under title:

Clinical reactions to food.

(A Wiley medical publication)
Includes index.
1. Food allergy.   2. Nutritionally induced diseases.
I. Lessof, M. H.   II. Series.
RC596.C54   1983   616.97′5   82-11101

ISBN 0 471 10436 1

British Library Cataloguing in Publication Data:

Clinical reactions to food.
1. Food allergy
I. Lessof, M. H.
616.97′5   RC596

ISBN 0 471 10436 1

Phototypeset by Dobbie Typesetting Service, Plymouth, Devon
Printed by Page Brothers Limited, Norwich, Norfolk

List of Contributors

R. StC. Barnetson   *Consultant Dermatologist and Senior Lecturer, Department of Dermatology, The Royal Infirmary, Edinburgh*

W. T. Cooke   *Honorary Consultant Physician and Gastroenterologist, The General Hospital, Birmingham.*

A. Ferguson   *Reader in Medicine, Gastrointestinal Unit, Western General Hospital, Crewe Road, Edinburgh.*

E. Hanington   *Honorary Consultant, Princess Margaret Migraine Clinic, Charing Cross Hospital, London, and City of London Migraine Clinic.*

G. K. T. Holmes   *Consultant Physician and Gastroenterologist, The Derbyshire Royal Infirmary, Derby, and Clinical Tutor, The University of Nottingham, Nottingham.*

J. H. Lacey   *Senior Lecturer and Hon. Consultant, Academic Department of Psychiatry, Jenner Wing, St. George's Hospital Medical School, London.*

M. H. Lessof   *Professor of Medicine, Guy's Hospital Medical School, London.*

I. Macdonald   *Professor of Applied Physiology, Guy's Hospital Medical School, London.*

D. A. Moneret-Vautrin   *Professeur Agrégé, Médecine Interne et Immuno-Allergologie, C.H.U. de Brabois, Route de Neufchateau, Vandoevre-les-Nancy, France.*

J. Soothill   *Professor of Immunology, Institute of Child Health, 30 Guildford Street, London.*

Contents

Preface

Food allergy has, in the past, been variously regarded as part of fringe medicine or a kind of cult subject, attracting the attention of newspapers, television, and the more popular medical periodicals. Until now, there have been relatively few comments on the subject from the medical profession at large. As the evidence accumulates, however, clinical reactions to food — both allergic and non-allergic — are seen to be of considerable importance, and an objective examination of the problem is clearly needed. It is the object of this book to provide it.

The traditional allergists were the first to make clear observations about the recurrence of untoward reactions to food in sensitized individuals, but they left the scientific proof of their discoveries to another generation. Clinical ecologists have also campaigned for the problem to be given due prominence but have, at the same time, avoided the critical approach which can establish how much of the growing folklore on the subject is based on observation and how much is sheer speculation.

The authors who have written in this book on food intolerance have focused on a number of different aspects — immunological, clinical and psychological. Seen in these terms, it is clear that people who have symptoms of food intolerance should no longer be offered a crude approach to diagnosis and a blunderbuss approach to treatment. Whether they have enzyme defects, other causes of food idiosyncrasy, food allergy or psychological problems, those who react to foods of one kind or another deserve to have their problem examined carefully. This is a subject in which the separation of fact and fiction is long overdue.

January 1983   M. H. LESSOF

Clinical Reactions to Food
Edited by M. H. Lessof
© 1983 John Wiley & Sons Ltd.

Nutrition in the Western World

Ian Macdonald

Department of Physiology,
Guy's Hospital Medical School,
London

When you do not have any money the problem is food; when you
have money it is sex; when you have both it is health; and when
everything is simply great then you are frightened of death.
(From: *The Ginger Man*, by J. P. Donleavy)

Except for small isolated groups, the anxiety of the adult in the Western World
is not whether there is enough food for survival but whether he can indulge
himself in those foods whose organoleptic properties he finds so desirable, and
at the same time not risk a reduction of life-span or early onset of physical
disability. In the Third World the problem is a lack of food, in the Western
World the problem is a surfeit of food and this food is available at an
acceptable economic price. It is mainly with respect to the hazards of excess, or
the risks from the refining of food, that the nutrition of the Western World
has to be considered.

That there are hazards, in terms of morbidity and mortality, associated with
an excess of food cannot be denied. However, several self-styled 'authorities'
have taken on their shoulders the responsibility for warning their fellows in the
Western World of the theoretical dangers of other aspects of Western food.
Most of the evidence on which their warnings are based is through association
rather than through a cause-and-effect relationship. This type of association to
promote a belief is well seen in the bulk of the evidence put forward for the
consumption of more dietary 'fibre', where comparisons are made between
populations in the Western World and Third World countries. An equally
valid association, and logically just as unsound, would be to point out that the
populations of those countries with high 'fibre' intakes die at an earlier age
than those whose diet contains less fibre, and the uncharitable could therefore
conclude that dietary 'fibre' reduces the life-span.

On the other hand if no action were to be taken or advice given before a cause-and-effect relationship was scientifically proved then unnecessary disability would ensue. It is, therefore, not easy to decide what dietary advice should be given to the inhabitant of the Western World who wishes to indulge in the pleasures of a particular type of food. However, if the advice is to change the pattern of the diet or of eating, then it is imperative to know that the new regime is without risk, a risk that might indeed be greater than one that it is hoped to avoid.

The level of uncertainty about the diet in the Western World, and its role in inducing disease, is due to three major factors. One is the fact that the control system in any metabolic reaction may be set at different levels between individuals—as is seen, for example, in the fact that one person can eat large quantities of saturated fat with little effect on the serum cholesterol concentration whereas another person, with a smaller intake of such fat, would have a striking increase in the level of serum cholesterol. We do not all react in the same way to the same nutritional (or any other) stimulus and this variation in response is compounded by physiological variables such as age, sex, physical and mental activity.

Another factor that is responsible for the high level of uncertainty—and hence spawning speculation—is the difficulty of assessing all the variables in a person's life-style, thus making it difficult to pinpoint any particular item. An example of this problem is seen in the dramatic fall in the incidence of ischaemic heart disease that has taken place in the past decade or so in the USA. Is this fall due to a reduced intake of fat (and in particular saturated fat), or to more physical exercise (jogging) or to less smoking, or to an increased awareness to maintain normal weight? Whether it is one or more of these variables, or some other variable, that is responsible will never be known.

A third difficulty in the way of obtaining evidence to show a cause-and-effect relationship between nutritional intake and disease is the long latent period between the consumption of the substance in the diet and its undesirable consequences. The high incidence of atheroma in US personnel killed in Korea suggests that atheroma is laid down before the age of 20 years or so, whereas in Norway in World War II there seemed to be a very short latent period in that the incidence of ischaemic heart disease fell markedly during the period of food deprivation and much stress, and increased again as soon as food supplies became more normal.

Thus it can be realized that the sum of knowledge on the undesirable consequences of consuming food in the Western World is limited and imprecise. This shortage of facts is fodder for those who, for one reason or another, wish to speculate about the possible ills in the Western World accruing from consuming certain foods that are either plentiful and cheap or pleasurable when compared with those living in less privileged circumstances.

This chapter will be concerned with discussing in a scientific (or some might say iconoclastic) way some of the health problems of the Western World that have been associated with nutrition.

OVER-WEIGHT

There are no satisfactory definitions of either over-weight or obesity and these turns may well be synonymous. There is no shortage of attempts to define over-weight, from ratios based on weight and height, body density, Metropolitan Life Insurance Tables, isotopic measurement of body fat, skin-fold thickness, clinical assessment, etc. Despite this failure to specify what is meant by over-weight it is confidently stated that 20 per cent of adults in the UK are over-weight and one-third in the USA are more than 20 per cent over 'ideal weight'. It has been stated that being over-weight is the commonest form of malnutrition in the Western World.

Disadvantages of being over-weight

Degenerative disease in the joints from increased weight-bearing is accepted as being a hazard of being over-weight, but the suggestion that respiratory problems are more common in the over-weight does not have conclusive evidence to support it, as the respiratory response to weight loss in the over-weight is variable. Due to the increase in cardiac output which is necessary when over-weight, the size of the heart is increased, as in an athlete who also demands greater cardiac output. Hypertension may also be more frequent in the over-weight and contributes to cardiomegaly; and a loss in weight is frequently associated with a fall in blood pressure.

The association between over-weight and diabetes with its complications is widely accepted though, of course, the insulin levels in these people are higher than in normal-weight individuals. One of the complications of diabetes is cardiovascular disease, but the evidence that the over-weight have a greater incidence of cardiovascular disease is not clear. What is certain is that coronary disease in an over-weight person is more likely to have a fatal outcome because of the increased cardiac demands, even at rest, in an over-weight person.

The psychological stresses of over-weight are well known. Whether these are *propter hoc* or *post hoc* may vary from person to person, but it seems that many of the psychological problems arise from the social mores of the community. The paintings of Hogarth (1698–1764) tell us how different is the social approach to over-weight now, as compared to the eighteenth century, and in some communities to be over-weight is an outward and visible sign of success and affluence.

Advantages of being over-weight

It has been suggested that being over-weight is part of evolution, in that in times of plenty body fat is laid down. Should food become scarce the over-weight individuals will be the most likely to survive. There is evidence to back this hypothesis in that epidemiological studies suggest decreased mortality in the obese, and that fat people survive better with malignancy and tuberculosis.

Possible underlying metabolic disorders in the over-weight

It is currently assumed that over-weight is not the norm — though with such a large proportion of over-weight adults in the Western World, the so-called presently considered 'normal' weight of the body will, in a decade or so, become subnormal, and will need to be re-named as 'desirable' body weight with a new set of criteria for defining the word 'desirable'. It is necessary to ask in what way the metabolic processes of the over-weight differ from those of lesser weight, apart that is, from the altered metabolism brought about by the increased amount of adipose tissue *per se*; and is it an alteration in the rate of metabolic processes that leads to over-weight and not vice-versa?

In an attempt to explain why thin people seem to eat large amounts of food and stay thin, whereas the reverse seems to be so in the over-weight, two hypotheses that need to be studied seriously have recently been advanced.

In one the hypothesis is that there exists in the breakdown of molecules such as, for example, glucose, a *'futile cycle'*. This means that when a molecule is partially broken down, in maybe the liver, it is immediately re-synthesized and this requires energy. The molecule is then broken down again and again re-synthesized and so on. Instead of the molecule completing its breakdown to its end-products with maximum efficiency, recycling of the intermediate products is less efficient.

That the 'futile cycle' exists in nature is not in dispute and the excess heat produced by 'futile cycles' is used, for example, by the bee to raise its body temperature in order that its metabolism can proceed rapidly enough to provide energy for it to fly. It has also been noted that some pigs seem to have more 'futile cycle' activity than others and are more liable to die of hyperthermia as a result.

Attempts to support this hypothesis in man are obviously not easy because it is difficult to eliminate such variables as thyroid and catecholamine output, for example, both of which may vary the resting metabolic rate (energy output at rest) and hence alter the efficiency of the body in terms of the proportion of energy in food which is used for body energy, rather than being wasted as excess heat.

Further development of the theme that over-weight persons may be more efficient in handling the energy consumed in food has been the recent renewed interest in '*brown fat*'. The young of many species, including man, have small areas of adipose tissue which appear more brown in colour than the surrounding yellow adipose tissue and these areas seem to be localized to certain regions, such as, for example, the scapular area. The brown appearance of the 'brown fat' may be due to its comparatively rich blood supply, and it also has a rich sympathetic nerve supply and the individual cells have an increased number of mitochondria.

The presumed physiological role of 'brown fat' in infants is that when threatened by a fall in body temperature, sympathetic nerve impulses to the 'brown fat' increase and these increase considerably the breakdown of energy by the mitochondria in each 'brown fat' cell, and the increased production of heat tends to offset any fall in body temperature.

As far as the over-weight person is concerned it is proposed that he or she has less 'brown fat' in adulthood than the normal weight individual and is thus less likely to burn off as much energy from food.

Evidence to support this hypothesis in over-weight adults is limited, and though the hypothesis cannot be rejected at this stage as a cause for over-weight, it should not encourage the complacent over-weight person from ceasing to try to lose weight because 'it's my glands'.

In conclusion it may be stated that if over-weight in the Western World is considered to be undesirable, for whatever reasons, then the metabolic cause underlying being over-weight should be established and treatment directed at the cause. If, as has been suggested, over-weight is an evolutionary advance, to prepare for times of scarcity, then the over-weight will have to voluntarily face periods of reduced energy intake.

'THE SACCHARINE DISEASES'

In 1966 a small book was first published by Cleave with the basic theme that the food, and particularly the carbohydrate-containing food, eaten in the Western World was too refined. The implication was that in the process of refining the food some nutritionally desirable components had been removed and it was the removal of these components that accounted for the increased incidence of certain diseases in the Western World, when compared with less industrialized countries. Though the book, and subsequent editions, was thin in scientifically acceptable cause-and-effect data, the concept was to give rise to considerable interest and new thinking about the role of those diseases thought to be due to 'nutritional abundance'. It was perhaps the first time that serious thought had been given to a possible harmful role of modern food, the Western World having, until less than 50 years earlier, been more concerned with nutritional deprivation and therefore not having concerned itself unduly with the consequences of modern methods for modifying food.

From this book by Cleave, which must surely be a landmark in nutritional thinking, much of what is discussed later stems.

FIBRE

Currently perhaps the most fashionable item in the diet considered to be of widespread benefit to the population at large is in fact not a nutrient at all, and is referred to as dietary fibre. The term fibre, like vitamin, refers to various substances with one feature in common. The common feature about dietary fibre is that it is not digested by the gut enzymes and is mainly composed of plant cell wall. A precise definition of various fibres is awaited, and, with the exception of lignin, dietary fibre is made up of carbohydrates. In view of the diversity of composition it is perhaps not surprising that various claims have been made for its value in the prevention and treatment of disease, and moreover many of the claims are based on association and hence are ill-founded. Perhaps the strangest aspect of the fibre story is that an article in the food that has no nutritional role is considered to be so important in our well-being.

When the excitement and enthusiasm for dietary fibre are over and less emotional judgements prevail it may be found that its value, both prophy-lactically and therapeutically, is more limited than current suppositions would lead one to believe.

Perhaps the first perceived claim for dietary fibre was that it was a 'must' in the treatment of diverticular disease of the colon. This represented a complete reversal of the previous low-residue diet that had been advocated for this condition, and there seemed no doubt that patients with diverticular disease had less discomfort on a high-fibre diet. Whether a high-fibre diet is of other than 'placebo' value in this condition has recently been queried. The fibre enthusiasts, some of whom displayed an almost missionary zeal, then hypothesized that fibre prevents diverticulosis, using the logic that if aspirin cures headache then an absence of aspirin causes headache. There is as yet no convincing evidence to allow one to conclude that a diet low in fibre is a factor in the aetiology of diverticulosis.

Related to its role in the treatment of diverticulosis is the fact that certain dietary fibres decrease intestinal transit time, the commonest fibre in this respect being wheat bran. It is beyond doubt that the consistency and volume of the stool is altered by bran and that it has a part to play in the treatment of mild constipation. It has even been stated, with some authority, that bran not only decreases transit time in the constipated, but increases it in those with diarrhoea! What has been assumed in all these studies is that a decrease in intestinal time in Western man/woman is desirable. In fact there is evidence to suggest that the hurry induced by bran may prevent the absorption of some nutrients, and could therefore be less than desirable.

Again linked with this one effect of bran, that each person can experience himself, is the suggestion that in the absence of dietary fibre the delay in the passage of gut contents allows bile salts to linger in the colon for a sufficient length of time to be converted by the gut bacteria to carcinogens and hence a bran-poor diet may result in carcinoma of the colon. Despite the attractiveness of this hypothesis in a disease of increasing prevalence in the Western World, there is no hard evidence as yet to support it.

Turning now to the higher reaches of the gut there is quite a large amount of evidence accumulating to support the view that certain fibres in the diet, namely pectin and guar gum, can be of value in the treatment of diabetes mellitus. When glucose is accompanied by either of these gums the ensuing blood glucose levels and insulin concentrations are lower than when the glucose is given alone. Reports talk of reduced therapeutic insulin in diabetics taking guar or pectin, and obviously this would appear to be an area of usefulness of dietary fibre that could make a clinical impact.

That dietary fibre prevents or delays the onset of atherosclerosis and coronary artery disease is a predictable claim that has been made. Pectin and to some extent guar slightly lower the serum cholesterol concentration, though there is no evidence to link the commonest disease of the Western World with the refining of the food.

In the heady excitement and hope that followed on the fibre concept its disadvantages were rather neglected. Children in the Third World are more prone to intestinal volvulus and intussuspection than Western children, and Burkitt is of the opinion that this is due to the greater content of fibre in the diet of Third World children. Various types of fibre, notably bran, contain phytate which combines with divalent cations such as iron, calcium, zinc, magnesium and phosphorus, and deficiencies of these elements in children due to dietary bran have been reported. It has also been reported that bran contains a trypsin inhibitor, and the loss of dietary protein which this may engender may be of some significance in Third World populations on a marginal protein intake.

Most of the prophylactic and therapeutic claims made for dietary fibre may well be wishful thinking. However, in the process of testing these ideas and hopes, much has been and will be learnt which is of value to the well-being of the Western World, and hopefully the Third World. The current view of an expert UK committee is that we should eat more dietary fibre, because it is unlikely to be harmful and could well be beneficial.

'NATURAL FOODS'

Part of the popular appear of dietary fibre is based on the notion that food in the Western World is too refined, and therefore there has been a swing to the other extreme; namely the belief that food that has not been processed and that has been grown without the addition of any substance by man, would be more health-giving than the regular Western food. Hence the terms 'natural', 'organic', and 'health' foods. This concept can be practised by only a few in the Western World, because added fertilizers, pesticides and refining not only make food cheaper but more plentiful, so in their absence only the more wealthy could afford the increased cost of 'natural' foods and not suffer from deficiency states.

There are in fact, dangers from consuming 'natural' foods, partly because they are exempt from the industrial standards. It has also been reported that raw milk can give rise to salmonella-associated illnesses; herb and other such teas and infusions may contain toxic products; and lead and other trace metal poisoning can occur after excessive consumption of bone meal, given as a source of calcium. The complete lack of any scientific rationale behind the urge to consume more 'natural' foods shows how emotional ('natural is better') is the judgement many make regarding food. What is perhaps more surprising is that despite emotional judgements, and with little in the way of nutritional education, nutritional deficiency states are very rarely seen in the Western World. Education in nutrition in the Western World should perhaps be more concerned with how to prevent excesses, rather than with how to avoid deficiencies.

FAST FOODS AND SNACKS

There is a tendency for more people, especially in early adulthood, to eat a rapid meal away from the home or to bring home food that has been prepared and cooked outside. For a variety of reasons, the pattern of eating in the UK is moving away from the traditional meal of meat or fish and two vegetables eaten at home, and this change in eating pattern needs to be considered from the nutritional aspect. All food must meet two fundamental requirements, namely adequacy—in terms of energy intake, and variety—to meet the need for proteins, vitamins, minerals, etc. As long as these are met by food, however taken, then the diet will be satisfactory. 'Fast' food and snacks are quite capable of fulfilling these requirements, and so long as the basic tenets of nutritional requirements are followed, the move away from the 'traditional' meal need not necessarily be accompanied by malnutrition.

Part of the apparent desire to spend less time on preparing and eating food is seen in the change in the breakfast pattern in the UK, where a recent survey showed that only 18 per cent of men, women and children eat a cooked breakfast, with 40 per cent eating a cereal-based breakfast. It has been suggested that this change may lead to undesirable effects, not so much on the nutrition of the individual but on his performance. In children who had omitted breakfast physical performance, as well as learning ability, was reduced during the morning as compared with controls. It has also been suggested, but not proven, that road accidents in the morning which involve only one vehicle may be due to the reactive hypoglycaemia of the driver who has had a hasty hot drink with ample sugar and no other food before starting the journey. It has also been reported that a glucose-containing drink given in the morning to steel-workers reduced the accident rate compared to controls.

'Junk' food is a term which the users cannot define and which is a contradiction in terms. No food is junk, as all food contains nutrients; and no one food contains all the substances necessary for healthy living—even breast milk is deficient in iron.

SUGGESTED NEW FUNCTIONS OF VITAMINS

It was the discovery of vitamins a century or so ago that led many people to consider that malnutrition was simply a deficiency problem that could be righted by taking a pill. To some extent this concept still prevails. This is to the detriment of the wider role that nutrition plays in preventing disease and to the encouragement of those who might wish to capitalize on this outdated concept.

The practitioners of fringe medicine in the Western World have long advocated the use of various patent preparations containing essential nutrients, in varying amounts and proportions, as a panacea for various specific diseases and disorders. This approach, whose main benefit was presumably psychological (because no evidence was available to support any physical merits) received considerable support from a scientist of international repute who had received Nobel Prizes for Physics and Peace. Dr Pauling turned his outstanding talents to a consideration of the value of ascorbic acid (vitamin C) as a prophylactic agent, in such large amounts that they were subsequently labelled megadoses. Quite an amount of research has been carried out to test the validity of these claims, in particular the ability of large doses of vitamin C in the prevention of the common cold, with mixed results. With reference to the common cold the Department of Drugs of the American Medical Association in 1975 concluded that concerning ascorbic medication:

(1) there is 'little convincing evidence to support claims of clinically important efficacy';
(2) 'we cannot advocate its unrestricted use for such purposes';

and a more recent review by the British Nutrition Foundation in general reinforces these views.

It is well recognized that large doses of fat-soluble vitamins can be harmful because the body has no rapid method of eliminating fats, whereas water-soluble vitamins in excess can be excreted in the urine. However, when doses greater than 100 times the daily requirement are consumed—as is advocated with vitamin C—some doubt must be case as to the body's ability to eliminate such excesses, and there are reports of headache, nausea, and blurred vision due to megadoses of vitamin C. It has been suggested that megadoses of ascorbic acid give rise to renal calculi, gastrointestinal disturbances and a conditioned need for ascorbic acid.

Vitamin E, for long considered to be a 'vitamin in search of a disease', is, without doubt, a true vitamin in man, mainly in premature infants where a deficiency gives rise to anaemia. A deficiency in adults is very difficult to produce. However, vitamin E has, in the opinion of large numbers of people in the Western World, properties wider than those even hinted at experimentally. These include longevity and prevention of scar tissue after operation. As vitamin E is fat-soluble the strictures that apply to any large doses of such vitamins apply, but seemingly no specific symptoms or signs apart from nausea and intestinal discomfort have been reported from its large-scale use, by mouth, in man. The widespread application of vitamin E to the skin is less likely to be of danger because little would be absorbed.

A suggested role for vitamin E that has scientific logic, though lacking in evidence, is that increased amounts of vitamin E should accompany an increased intake of polyunsaturated fatty acids. The rationale behind this is that the double-bonds in a polyunsaturated fatty acid are unstable and may take up oxygen readily with the formation of potential carcinogens. As vitamin E is an anti-oxidant this process of oxygen uptake by the double-bonds in the polyunsaturated fat molecule would be inhibited. A logical story with, as yet, no basis in fact.

From time to time various new so-called 'vitamins' are reported in the lay press but are not worthy of consideration here.

The promotion and sale of nutritional supplements is a growing and profitable business in the Western World, and though some of the products are well formulated and contain balanced amounts of vitamins and minerals, some contain megadoses of single nutrients, compounds with no established nutritional function such as vitamin B_{17}, vitamin P, hesperidin, and RNA. Use of such supplements may induce a false sense of complacency and a lack of interest in choosing a nutritionally sound diet. Since they also allow for a possible combination of supplements to produce undesirable nutrient interactions or nutritional imbalances, they are obviously to be discouraged.

FOOD ADDITIVES

Food in the Western World is characterized by having added to it substances which help to preserve it by increasing shelf-life, substances which add or enhance flavour, substances which help to maintain the appearance a consumer expects (e.g. keeping canned peas green), etc. By increasing shelf-life the additive is not only ensuring that its consumption will not result in clinical disorder, but because it can be kept longer and still be safe to eat the food is cheaper. The principle of adding substances to preserve food has been practised for millennia. The addition of substances for organoleptic purposes is, perhaps, not so directly desirable but if the additive in the amounts used is harmless then its use for this purpose seems justifiable.

The large choice of foods throughout the year at acceptable costs has been made possible in the Western World by two important aspects of food science, one by the addition of chemical substances, and the other by freezing the food. The former is controversial and not unreasonably so as any addition to food should make it safer, not the reverse. The rapid freezing of fresh food not only inhibits microbiological growth multiplication but in many cases preserves the high level of a food component which would otherwise be reduced were the food not so preserved (e.g. ascorbic acid in frozen peas).

It must be accepted (see Chapter 6) that unpleasant reactions to food additives do occur, and that a minority of the population are capable of developing allergic or other adverse reactions to processed or, indeed, to 'natural' foods. However, this hazard needs to be kept in perspective. The frequently expressed judgements that food additives should not be allowed should be balanced against the risks that are found in unprocessed foods such as cabbage, broad beans, potatoes, rhubarb and home-made jam. Unlike additives, natural foods are not extensively tested and yet have the reputation of being 'pure' and in every way beneficial to health. It has recently been stated, with evidence to support it, that 'of the potential sources of harm in foods the largest by far are first microbiological contamination and next, nutritional imbalance. Risks from environmental contamination are about 1000 times less and risk from pesticide residues and food additives can be estimated as about 100 times smaller again. Naturally occurring compounds in food are more likely to cause toxicity than intentional food additives' (See Coppock, 1979).

FOOD AND CANCER

As discussed earlier, much has been written recently about dietary fibre and colon cancer, and also about dietary saturated fats and breast cancer. It therefore comes as somewhat of a surprise to learn that there is a hypothesis that certain foods may *prevent* cancer and that this hypothesis has some acceptable scientific evidence to support it. 'Every year there are 125,000 deaths from cancer in England and it seems ironic that one of the most promising cancer preventative agents to come from several decades and hundreds of million of pounds spent on cancer research should be a long-known essential nutrient' (Buckley, 1981). This substance is vitamin A (retinol) and its analogues.

It has been found in animals that the amount of vitamin A in the diet has a marked inverse effect on the effectiveness of many carcinogens but in man the evidence is, at the moment, limited largely to retrospective studies of vitamin A intake. Serum vitamin A levels have been shown to be lower in cancer patients than in controls, even before they developed cancer.

SALT AND ARTERIAL HYPERTENSION

A role for dietary sodium in the pathogenesis of hypertension is not a new hypothesis, and there is much to support this hypothesis from various areas of the world, though it is not entirely clear whether the hypertension results from an increase in the intake of sodium or a concomitant decrease in potassium ingestion. Current thinking is that there is an at-risk group in the population and that perhaps prophylactic dietary advice concerning a reduced sodium intake needs to be given to this group only. It is too early to define precisely the role of dietary sodium and potassium, or perhaps the ratio of these two in food. Such studies as have been carried out on the treatment, as opposed to the prevention, of hypertension — a condition that seems to be common in the Western World — would suggest that a reduced sodium intake is an important part of therapy.

FOOD AND CORONARY HEART DISEASE

The literature, both lay and professional, contains reports that place the blame for the increased incidence of coronary artery disease (CHD) on certain constituents of the diet. Fats, carbohydrates, and some amino acids have variously been blamed for the increase in incidence of CHD, and this fact alone suggests that no one dietary item is responsible. This does not necessarily exclude diet as an aetiological factor because there is evidence to suggest that at least two metabolic disturbances are associated with CHD and that for each disorder a different diet should be prescribed. For example it has been suggested that those persons with a raised serum cholesterol concentration should reduce their intake of saturated fat in order to achieve a fall in the serum cholesterol level, but whether this fall in serum cholesterol is beneficial in avoiding or prolonging the CHD event is less certain. On the other hand it was suggested that an increase in the level of triglycerides in fasting serum might be a predictor of CHD, and evidence exists to show that a reduced intake of dietary carbohydrate reduces the fasting serum triglyceride level. The lack of any conclusive evidence involving diet in CHD must, to some extent, be due to the variation in the metabolism of the potential CHD population. Also in any prospective study at least 60 per cent are not going to get CHD, even if they are males over 35 years old. Women before the menopause, whether natural or artificial, are not at such great risk.

More recently evidence has been accumulating to suggest that the total level of serum cholesterol is less valuable as an indicator of future CHD than the high-density lipoprotein fraction of the cholesterol (HDL cholesterol). If this is so it might be considered desirable to *raise* this fraction (the higher the level the less the risk of CHD) by dietary means. Little is known at the moment about how this could be achieved, though it is possible that a moderate alcohol intake, and perhaps an increase in chromium in the diet, will raise the level.

What is perhaps not sufficiently appreciated is that it may not be the cholesterol in the serum that is a factor in the causation of CHD but that raised cholesterol, in whatever form, may be just one feature of the process that leads to CHD. Taking steps to reduce it can be likened to cutting merely a branch, when it is desired to cut down the whole tree.

Many official bodies from various parts of the world have looked critically at the role of diet in preventing CHD and have offered appropriate advice. In the main their advice is to cut down on fat intake, especially saturated fat, and to eat more complex carbohydrates. A reduction in sugar intake is frequently also recommended but the evidence to support this is very flimsy. More recently a 'middle of the road' view has been published in the USA which supports the concept of moderation in the articles of food eaten. When advising whole populations or communities there is, of course, the moral dilemma of whether to advise the reduction of an article of the diet that may give much gustatory pleasure, when only a minority are going to benefit from this advice. Perhaps the answer may lie in learning what factor in the blood is involved directly with CHD (if any is) and then giving the appropriate dietary advice to those who, on blood examination of the whole population at regular intervals, are found to have the abnormality.

CONCLUSION

In the Western World the food we eat is determined less by physiological demands than by gustatory wishes and, among some, the feeling that certain foods are 'good' or 'bad' for health. This being so, judgements on the health value of a food in terms of promoting or preventing disease are influenced largely by emotion, with the argument that 'I am alive and well and therefore the diet I eat must be correct'. This view is patently false but does lead those who have the welfare of their fellows at heart to make pronouncements which the media are happy to promulgate because they are newsworthy. Some of these pronouncements are non-scientific, and turn out to be nonsense.

FURTHER READING AND REFERENCES

Over-weight

Bray, G. A. (1976). The overweight patient. *Adv. Int. Med.*, **21**, 267–308.
Fitzgerald, F. T. (1981). The problem of obesity. *Ann. Rev. Med.*, **32**, 221–31.
Foster, D. O., and Frydman, M. L. (1978). Non-shivering thermogenesis in the rat. *Can. J. Physiol. Pharmacol.*, **56**, 110–22.
Garrow, J. S. (1974). *Energy Balance and Obesity in Man*. North Holland Publishing Co., London.

James, W. P. T., and Trayhurn, P. (1976). An integrated view of the metabolic and genetic basis for obesity. *Lancet*, **2**, 770-2.

Saccharine diseases

Cleave, T. L. (1974). *The Saccharine Disease*. John Wright & Sons, Bristol.

Fibre

Anderson, J. W. (1980). Dietary fibre and diabetes. In: *Medical Aspects of Dietary Fiber* (Eds G. A. Spiller and R. M. Kay). Plenum Medical, London.
Burkitt, D. P., and Trowell, H. C. (1975). *Refined Carbohydrate Foods and Disease*. Academic Press, London.
Mendeloff, A. I. (1976). Dietary fibre. In: *Present Knowledge in Nutrition*, pp.392-401. Nutrition Foundation, New York, Inc., Washington.
Royal College of Physicians (1980). *Medical Aspects of Dietary Fibre*. Pitman Medical, London.

Fast foods and snacks

British Nutrition Foundation (1981). Snack meals—trends and effects. *Nutr. Bull.*, **16**, 43-8.

Suggested new functions of vitamins

Hughes, R. E. (1981). *Vitamin C: Some Current Problems*. British Nutrition Foundation, London.
National Nutritional Consortium Inc. (1979). *Vitamin-Mineral Safety, Toxicity and Misuse*. American Dietetic Association, Chicago.
Present Knowledge in Nutrition (1976). Various articles on vitamins, pp.64-231. Nutrition Foundation, New York Inc., Washington.

Food additives

Why Additives (1977). Forbes, London.
Coppock, J. B. M. (1979). Natural toxicants and food additives. *Br. Nutrition Found. Bull.*, **5**, 145-52.

Food and cancer

Buckley, J. D. (1981). Vitamin A and the prevention of cancer. *Br. Nutr. Found. Bull.*, **6**, 142-52.
Kark, J. D., Smith, A. H., and Hames, C. G. (1982). Serum retinol and the inverse relationship between serum cholesterol and cancer. *Br. Med. J.*, **1**, 152-4.

Salt and arterial hypertension

Williams, D. R. R. (1980). Salt intake and the pathogenesis of hypertension. *Br. Nutr. Found. Bull.*, **5**, 187-93.

Food and coronary heart disease

Eating for Health. (1978). DHSS; HMSO, London.
Towards Healthful Diets. (1980). National Research Council; Nat. Acad. Sc., US, Washington.

Clinical Reactions to Food
Edited by M. H. Lessof
© 1983 John Wiley & Sons Ltd and M. H. Lessof

Challenges to Medical Orthodoxy

R. StC. Barnetson and M. H. Lessof

*The Royal Infirmary, Edinburgh,
and Guy's Hospital, London*

Introduction

A recent leader in the *Lancet* (1982) on 'Food allergy and intolerance' began as follows:

> Nobody doubts that food allergy exists but the subject has acquired a dubious reputation. One reason is that the diagnosis has been overworked to explain a great array of poorly understood clinical symptoms. Extravagent therapeutic claims have excited an antagonistic response, putting the subject under a cloud of controversy (which perhaps shelters a little quackery).

These few sentences summarize succinctly the present situation regarding food allergy, as viewed by the medical profession.

It is now recognized that ingestion of foods may result in clinical manifestations due to a number of different mechanisms, and the term 'allergy' is unfortunately viewed differently by the ecologist and the clinical immunologist. Herein lies the crux of the problem. The word allergy was coined by von Pirquet (1906) who defined the phenomenon as an acquired specific altered capacity to react to physical substances on the part of the tissues of the body. This was necessarily a rather broad definition, and most physicians and scientists now reserve the term for phenomena resulting from immunological hypersensitivity, particularly that mediated by immunoglobulin E (IgE). Thus whereas only a few clinical manifestations may be attributed to IgE-mediated food allergy, as described by Lessof *et al.* (1980), most books on ecology describe food allergy as any adverse effect experienced by the patient as a result of ingesting a food.

The mechanisms by which foods may result in clinical symptoms may be summarized as follows:

(1) *The patient may be intolerant to a food* because it contains:
  (a) substances which themselves have a pharmacological action, e.g. histamine in fish such as mackerel, canned foods; tyramine in certain cheeses; caffeine;
  (b) substances which release chemical mediators, e.g. histamine released by tomatoes, strawberries;
  (c) substances which are toxic, e.g. hexachlorobenzene used as a dressing for seed wheat in Turkey resulting in acquired porphyria (Cam and Nigogosyan, 1963); acetanilide in rape-seed oil resulting in pneumono-pathy and respiratory failure (Tabuenca, 1981);
  (d) substances which are irritant to the intestinal mucosa, particularly if it is already diseased, e.g. highly spiced curries.
(2) *The patient may have idiosyncrasy to a food* because his intestine is deficient in important enzymes normally responsible for digestion of that food, e.g. lactase deficiency which results in diarrhoea when foods containing milk are ingested.
(3) *The patient may be truly allergic to a food*, with evidence of immuno-logical hypersensitivity. Compared with the other types of food in-tolerance, this is a comparatively rare event. Usually it is IgE-mediated, but a number of physicians and immunologists also include diseases which may be due to other sensitivity mechanisms within the Coombs and Gell classification (Coombs and Gell, 1963). Because a number of physicians and immunologists reserve the term 'allergy' for IgE-mediated hyper-sensitivity the term 'food-allergic disease' is now preferred, to cover all diseases due to hypersensitivity phenomena.

One other concept which should be mentioned is that of the 'masking of food allergy'. It is obvious that food allergy and intolerance might not be recognized, particularly if the food was a daily component of the diet. However Rinkel (1944) has suggested that some patients actually feel better after ingestion of the offending food, and symptoms may be delayed for 2–3 days: the validity of this concept remains open to question.

BACK TO NATURE AND ECOLOGY

It is probably fair to say that there are two main groups of people who are interested in adverse reactions to foods: the ecologists and the allergists. Whereas the Ecology Movement, as a whole, is concerned with the larger issues of man, his environment, and the damaging changes produced by modern living, the clinical ecologists are concerned with the pollutants in the atmosphere and in our drinking water and food, together with the health problems which these contaminants can cause. They have pressed for a more rigorous control of atmospheric pollution, better standards which prevent the contamination of food, and a more restricted use of food additives. Although they have received little acknowledgement, many of their ideas have been so widely adopted as to become commonplace.

Having drawn attention to the problems caused by pollution and contamination, the clinical ecologists now face a dilemma. In a scientific world it may not be sufficient to promulgate ideas without some proof of their validity. Like clinical allergists before them, the ecologists are now being pressed either to produce evidence for their claims, particularly where they concern medical treatment, or to withdraw. Whereas allergists, in a similar position, have accepted this challenge, ecologists have not always done so. A number of their claims remain unsubstantiated or, in some cases, have been exploited commercially by people who may be less well motivated than the ecologists themselves. Both the positive and negative aspects of the ecological approach therefore need to be considered.

It is undoubtedly true that the habitat of man in industrialized countries has changed very significantly over the past million years. Man was originally a herbivore, and in some parts of the world such as Kenya he remains so. However, comparatively recently in human evolution he has become an omnivore, and most people in the Western World and in the Far East have an extremely varied diet comprising many foods which are potential pharmacological agents, irritants, or allergens. The problem is compounded by the fact that foods are now preserved for considerable periods by processes such as canning, and it is therefore necessary to add preservatives and colouring agents which may themselves cause clinical manifestations (e.g. urticaria, abdominal pains).

There are now a very considerable number of books on the subject of 'food allergy' written by ecologists-cum-allergists. Most emanate from the USA and examples which immediately come to mind are those by A. H. Rowe (1931), A. F. Coca (1942), H. J. Rinkel, T. G. Randolph, and M. Zeller (1951) and latterly L. D. Dickey (1976). In the UK probably the best-known clinical ecologist is R. Mackarness whose books, *Not all in the Mind* (1976) and *Chemical Victims* (1980), present a disturbing but superficial outline of the problems of ecology in the modern world. Both books are intended for the lay reader and are uncritical in their approach, tending to quote case histories of patients whose clinical manifestations have been ameliorated by elimination of foods or by bizarre diets; both tend to the sensational, one cover proclaiming that the book is a 'revolutionary approach to the modern epidemics: allergies, headaches, lethargy, obesity, bowel disturbances, depression and other mental illnesses'; the other 'a startling look at the threat to your health by chemicals in food and household products'. Few would disagree that certain pollutants in the atmosphere, water, or foods are potential dangers of modern existence, but this dramatization does not strengthen the case.

The argument for taking food contamination seriously is in fact a strong one. There are several instances where contaminated food has resulted in illness or death on an epidemic scale, and there is every reason to suspect that numerous instances of less severe illness have gone undetected. When the industrial contamination of the water in Minamata Bay caused the death of 35 people who ate mercury-contaminated fish, much effort was needed to identify the cause of the disaster. The same is true of the mass poisoning outbreaks, due to tricresyl phosphate, which have resulted from the contamination of cooking oil (Hunter, 1978). A celebrated outbreak of hepatitis at Epping resulted when small amounts of diaminodiphenyl methane penetrated some sacks of flour (Harrington and Waldron, 1981); and there have now been numerous reports on the 'toxic–allergic' syndrome caused by contaminated rape-seed oil (see Chapter 6). Where the toxic effects of ingested substances is suspected, it is clearly not possible to investigate all unexplained symptoms; and where the symptoms are mild their cause may come to be detected almost by accident. An example may be given in the skin-sensitizing effect of the psoralens, which are present in several foods and drugs as well as in sunscreen lotions and which can lead to a persistent 'light reaction' long after the sensitizing material has been eliminated. There is thus ample evidence that clinical disease, both major and minor, can be transmitted by various foods. The examples given can only represent the tip of a very large iceberg.

By emphasizing the diseases which stem from our industrialized society, clinical ecologists have certainly made a contribution which has yet to be fully appreciated. Probably the main criticism that can be levelled at their efforts concerns their approach to the individual patient, whose symptoms may be attributed to 'food allergy' in the absence of any objective diagnostic criteria, or who may be treated empirically by methods which they believe to be effective but which have never been validated by any objective assessment.

Distinctions between food allergy, intolerance, and idiosyncrasy have yet to be integrated into the clinical ecologist's approach, and the published work on the subject tends to report individual case histories rather than to analyse the findings and the results in a series of patients. Without diagnostic criteria, without epidemiological studies to assess the nature and size of the problem, and without an objective assessment of the effects of treatment, the ecologist's approach has not yet evolved from the philosophical to the scientific. Even simple clinical observations are lacking—the proportion of patients with a certain clinical manifestation (e.g. arthritis, headache) in which food ingestion can be incriminated, or the mode of presentation which might lead the clinician to suspect food allergy or intolerance in the first instance. Much remains to be done, therefore, before the clinical validity of the ecologist's approach can be accepted.

DISEASES WHICH ARE CLAIMED TO BE FOOD-ALLERGIC: A CONTROVERSIAL ISSUE

There is still considerable controversy as to which conditions *are* definitely food-allergic diseases: most would agree that there are conditions where a direct causal relationship can be shown. Such diseases include rhinitis, conjunctivitis, asthma, atopic eczema, angioedema and urticaria, migraine, coeliac disease, and its variants such as dermatitis herpetiformis.

However even within this list there are difficulties. For instance, though some patients with atopic eczema have a definite history of food allergy with specific IgE to certain foods, this is by no means universal. Indeed, some patients may have classical atopic eczema with the classical history and clinical manifestations, although they have neither a history of inhalant or food allergy nor a raised IgE concentration to foods or inhalants. It might be argued on this basis that they are not atopic; yet it is also possible that they may have outgrown their allergies but persisted with their skin reactivity. Another disease on this list also gives rise to controversy: is coeliac disease due to hypersensitivity? Certainly there may be major immunological abnormalities (see Chapter 9), but there is an arguable case that gluten may be acting as a toxin rather than an allergen, particularly as it has been shown that normal subjects may develop jejunal mucosal changes if they ingest enough gluten (Doherty and Barry, 1981).

Apart from these examples there are a number of diseases where a food-allergic role has been suggested in the pathogenetic mechanism, but in most the case is far from proven. A number of conditions are due to the pharmacological effects of ingestants and represent food intolerance not food allergy, e.g. headache due to tyramine in canned fish, cardiac arrythmias due to caffeine. In yet other conditions it is still debated whether food allergy plays a role: they include rheumatoid arthritis, multiple sclerosis, ulcerative colitis, Crohn's disease, the 'total allergy syndrome', and hyperkinetic behaviour in childhood. Cot deaths in infancy were also suspected at one time of being due to milk allergy because of evidence based on animal studies which have not, however, been substantiated in man.

Rheumatoid arthritis

It has long been considered that food allergy may either cause or precipitate rheumatoid arthritis (RA), and there are various reasons for this. The American Arthritis Foundation however is in no doubt that there is *no* causal relationship between the two conditions. In a booklet entitled *Arthritis — The Basic Facts* the authors state quite categorically that, although some patients insist on believing that special diets are helpful in RA, the relationship between diet and RA has been thoroughly and scientifically studied with totally negative results—and that no food (or avoidance of food) is effective in treating or 'curing' it.

Despite this, there have been many publications documenting amelioration of the symptoms of patients with 'rheumatoid arthritis' following the avoidance of a food. However, it is important to realize that not everyone with 'arthritis' has rheumatoid arthritis. Gout could certainly respond to dietary restriction, and it is quite clear that a number of patients who are described as responding to diet have arthritis of non-rheumatoid type. In particular, it has been suggested that the well-recognized syndrome, 'palindromic rheumatism', is characterized by transient episodes of arthritis which may be related to food allergy. It is well recognized that when potential allergens are absorbed, circulating immune complexes are formed. In the right circumstances, it seems possible that arthritis could result and might lead to transient symptoms, rather than to the devastating permanent pathology which occurs in RA.

Many of the accounts in the older literature on rheumatoid arthritis are suspect because they are unsupported by adequate serological tests. This must include the book by Dong and Banks (1976) entitled *New Hope for the Arthritic*, which supports the idea that diet is useful in the treatment of RA. Although published recently, this describes the authors' experience over 37 years, but scientific and diagnostic data are inadequate and the progress of patients is described in the form of case reports. This criticism does not apply to a number of recent papers which have suggested that diet may influence the manifestations of patients with proven RA. Parke and Hughes (1981) described studies in one patient whose RA appeared to be exacerbated by the ingestion of dairy produce. On challenge with milk and cheese, this patient developed a pronounced increase in synovitis, which paralleled an increase in circulating immune complexes and increase in specific IgE antibodies to milk and cheese. Another recent paper by Sköldstram *et al.* (1979) also suggests that food avoidance may ameliorate the symptoms of RA, because they found that five of sixteen patients improved after fasting for 7–10 days, compared with only one of the ten RA controls who were not fasted. These two papers could suggest that further studies of the relationship between food ingestion and avoidance in RA might be fruitful.

It is certainly feasible, on theoretical grounds, that patients who have difficulty in clearing immune complexes from their bloodstream (because they suffer from RA) may have difficulty in handling the additional immune complexes which are known to be provoked by food (Paganelli *et al.*, 1979). This need not imply a causal relationship in the aetiology of RA *per se*.

In the context of food allergy, 'palindromic rheumatism' deserves further discussion, although it is probably unrelated to rheumatoid arthritis. This phenomenon was described by Solis-Cohen (1914), who wrote a paper entitled 'On some angioneural arthroses (periarthroses, pararthroses) commonly mistaken for gout or rheumatism'. Cohen described the appearance of painful swellings in joints or soft tissues, which occurred frequently at regular or irregular intervals (possibly daily, weekly, or less frequently), lasted a few hours to a few weeks, and then completely disappeared. It was given the name palindromic rheumatism by Hench and Rosenberg (1941), who studied 34 cases and suspected that in 16 'food allergy' was the cause of the exacerbations. No scientific evidence was offered for this view. Vaughan (1943) studied palindromic rheumatism among allergic persons and found that of 1000 'allergic' patients, 20 per cent complained of past or present joint pains or swelling and 3 per cent found that certain specified foods produced exacerbation or recurrence of rheumatic symptoms. Half of this group (27 patients) had positive skin tests to foods, and the other half had provocation of their symptoms following ingestion of the food. The foods implicated included pork, milk, eggs, tomatoes, strawberries, and other fruits. He concluded that food or inhalant allergy may be a cause of palindromic rheumatism, but it did not follow that it was the only cause.

Multiple sclerosis

The geographical incidence of multiple sclerosis (MS) varies very considerably from country to country. The view has been put forward that the geographical incidence may be related to diet. On the basis of epidemiological studies Shatin (1964) suggested that MS may be the result of gluten intolerance, and the view is still held by some that a gluten-free diet may be beneficial in this disease. However the studies of antibodies in MS by Wright *et al.* (1965) did not show that patients had high titres of gluten antibodies. They did show significantly raised titres of milk antibodies, and this has never been adequately explained.

A number of other studies are of historic rather than current interest. At least one epidemiological survey has suggested that diet may be important in the induction of MS (Swank, 1950) and biochemical studies have shown a deficiency of linoleate in the serum of MS patients (Baker *et al.*, 1964; Tichy *et al.*, 1969). A number of studies of linoleate supplementation of the diet have been carried out with varying results. Millar *et al.* (1973) showed that relapses were less severe and less frequent among those who took linoleate though there was no evidence of any change in the ultimate prognosis. Bates *et al.* (1978) did not find any difference in the frequency of exacerbations in patients who received a linoleic acid-supplemented diet, but relapses tended to be less severe in this group.

In summary, claims have been made that MS patients may be linoleate-deficient, but additions of linoleate to the diet have not resulted in a convincing amelioration of disease. None of these published reports suggests any evidence of immunological food allergy.

Ulcerative colitis and Crohn's disease

The aetiology of ulcerative colitis (UC) and Crohn's disease remains obscure. As in other conditions in which conventional medicine has provided an imperfect answer, food allergy has been considered as a causative factor. This theory was originally proposed by Andresen (1942) who felt that at least two-thirds of cases of UC were due to food allergy, a vast majority being due to milk allergy. Later Truelove (1961) described five patients with UC who were given a milk-free diet. When this was done, both their symptoms and the sigmoidoscopic appearances improved. Despite this interesting observation, milk-avoidance has not become part of the standard regime of therapy in UC. The possibility remains that secondary milk intolerance may occur in some cases of UC because of a loss of brush-border enzymes or for some other reason; but there is no evidence that milk acts as an allergen in such cases.

O'Morain *et al.* (1980) have used elemental diets in patients with Crohn's disease and found that in the majority, remissions of the disease resulted. The reason for this is unclear; although such a diet may be effective because it provides nutritional support or is hypoallergenic, it may also act as a medical bypass from the affected area or may alter bowel flora.

The total allergy syndrome

It has been suggested that extreme measures may sometimes be necessary to protect very sensitive individuals from exposure to the chemical contaminants in our industrial and domestic environment, including the petrol fumes and sulphur dioxide in the air we breathe, the artificial preservatives which contaminate our food and drink, and even the plasticizers which are present in tap water. Illogically, it is then suggested that patients who are so sensitive should be confined in an enclosed environment, receiving specially prepared food and breathing air which has been passed across industrial filters.

The concept of 'total allergy' has caught the imagination of many members of the public, who have been so concerned for the fate of people who are 'allergic to the twentieth century' that they have, in some instances, contributed generously towards the expensive treatment which has been offered to those who are suffering from this 'disease'. However, the criteria for making the diagnosis remain unclear. Reported symptoms include weakness, lethargy, faintness, convulsions, blackouts, anginal pain, asthma-like breathing, migraine, disorders of the bowel and bladder, aching joints, and cutaneous hypersensitivity. To these should be added the not uncommon symptoms of symmetrical paraesthesiae of the limbs, and muscle cramps — symptoms which can, in fact, be reproduced in susceptible subjects by 2 or 3 minutes of hyperventilation, leading to carbon dioxide loss and all the metabolic effects of hypocarbia (Nixon, 1982).

Extremely severe, multiple allergies can certainly occur—for example, in eosinophilic gastroenteritis (see Chapter 6)—but the criteria for diagnosing 'total allergy' do not suggest this condition and, indeed, have at no time been clearly defined in the medical press. As judged by attributed reports in the London *Observer* and *The Sunday Times*, they do not appear to require evidence of allergy or of gastrointestinal disease. It is perhaps a reflection of the trust which members of the public are prepared to place in newspaper and television reports—and their lack of trust in the medical profession—that there has nevertheless been some public pressure for units to be set up within the British National Health Service for the treatment of the victims of this disorder.

On the evidence which has so far become available, this diagnosis has sometimes been applied to hyperventilators, at other times to patients with anorexia nervosa or to hysterics. There is at present very little to suggest that the majority of patients who are so labelled have an allergic disease at all.

Allergy and psychiatric symptoms

It has been repeatedly suggested that either food-allergic reactions or some other form of food intolerance may be responsible for psychiatric symptoms which are by no means always accompanied by evidence of allergy in the conventional sense. Included in the wide range of symptoms which have been described are poor concentration, episodes of aggression, confusional states, and depression (Wraith, 1980). Some groups have noted a frequent association between psychiatric symptoms, headache, and migraine (Brown et al., 1981), without claiming that the symptoms have an immunological basis. In other studies (Rapp, 1978) it has been suggested that over two-thirds of children with the 'hyperkinetic syndrome' have clinical evidence of allergy in the form of nasal symptoms or skin reactions, and that a similar proportion have positive skin tests to 'dust and pollen' while 'appropriate skin test controls were negative'. Although publications on this subject may be open to criticism on methodological grounds, and because of the lack of detailed data, controlled studies have been reported in which psychiatric and other symptoms have been provoked by the offending food, given on a double-blind basis, both in adults (King, 1981; Brown et al., 1981) and in children with behaviour and learning problems attributed to the 'hyperkinetic syndrome' (Rapp, 1978, 1979; O'Shea and Porter, 1981). These reports are by no means generally accepted and not all authors have been able to provoke changes in behaviour by challenging with the supposedly offending substances (*Lancet*, 1982). Since there is, however, an occasional association between psychiatric problems and food reactions in such disorders as gluten enteropathy (see Chapter 9), these claims still require further investigation.

DIAGNOSTIC TESTS FOR DIAGNOSIS
OF FOOD ALLERGY AND INTOLERANCE

Another area of controversy surrounds the claims which have been made about tests used in the diagnosis of food allergy and intolerance. Some tests are of proven scientific value, whereas others are, at best, of doubtful validity. The former include the following:

(1) *Provocation tests* are of value, provided that they are carried out objectively. Patients who develop bizarre clinical manifestations when they are fed with a food in a recognizable form include malingerers, hyperventilators, and those who are psychiatrically ill. Tests should therefore be performed on a double-blind basis as far as possible, in order to avoid the misdiagnosis which may occur in functional states such as hysteria.

The hazards of open provocation are illustrated by a patient seen by Dr Parveen Kumar (personal communication), a child of 15 years who had complained of abdominal pains since the age of 7. At the age of 14 these became so severe that, according to her parents, they induced loss of consciousness for an hour. She had a considerable number of negative investigations, including skin-prick testing to a large battery of foods; but because she was reported to have serum gluten antibodies she was given a gluten-free diet — without benefit. She was therefore screened by electro encephalograph and electrocardiograph, given a disguised gluten challenge without ill effect and then given three small pieces of bread openly. Within 15 minutes she complained of abdominal pain, began to shout with pain after 30 minutes, and at that juncture appeared to lose consciousness (though she was rousable by painful stimuli). After a further 10 minutes she awoke and was emotionally labile. During the whole episode there was no electroencephalographic or electrocardiographic abnormality. A psychiatrist found her to have considerable emotional disturbance and concluded that her clinical manifestations were entirely hysterical.

It may be concluded that, although provocation tests are useful, the patient should not know which food is given. Observations should be reproducible and should not be induced by other foods. Even when they are positive, provocation tests do not necessarily differentiate between food allergy, food intolerance, and food idiosyncrasy.

(2) *Skin testing*. This is another area of controversy in the diagnosis of food allergy, since many allergists declare that prick tests and scratch tests are unhelpful. This may partly reflect the poor standardization of test extract but also the fact that a positive skin test can persist long after a childhood food allergy has subsided. Where well-defined positive (5 mm) skin tests to

food allergens correlate well with radio-allergosorbent tests, they appear to be useful in the diagnosis of IgE-mediated hypersensitivity. As might be expected, they are not helpful in other immunological types of hypersensitivity or in food intolerance not due to allergy. Reports of late skin reactions remain to be validated, including the claim that skin testing with gliadin in patients with coeliac disease can induce an Arthus-type or a delayed hypersensitivity reaction.

(3) *Radioallergosorbent tests* (RASTs) are useful in the diagnosis of food allergy but are expensive and may not be more informative than prick tests. The Pharmacia RAST is scored from 0 to 4, where a score of 4 may reflect 17.5->1000 RAST units (1 unit is roughly equivalent to 1 IU total IgE). While cross-reacting vegetable polysaccharides may have interfered with the specificity of this method in the past, improvements in methodology have made it possible for the RAST to become much more informative.

(4) *Assays of food antibodies other than IgE antibodies by precipitin, haemagglutination, or enzyme-linked immunosorbent assay tests.* These tests for IgG antibodies show a poor correlation with specific diseases but may be positive in gluten-sensitive enteropathy, perhaps because of increased intestinal permeability due to gut damage. Similar observations have been made in the past in ulcerative colitis (Jewell and Truelove, 1972).

(5) *Jejunal biopsies* demonstrate partial or subtotal villous atrophy in gluten-sensitive enteropathy. They are normal in patients with IgE-mediated food hypersensitivity (Braathen *et al.*, 1980; Barnetson *et al.*, 1981).

Tests used by allergists which are of more dubious value include the following:

(1) *The 'pulse test'.* This was first described by Coca (1942). There are a number of variations of this test, based on the claim that a 'food-allergic' patient may develop a significant rise in his heart rate following ingestion of a food to which he is intolerant. While supraventricular tachycardia may follow the ingestion of foods such as those containing caffeine, or may accompany other features of anaphylaxis, there is little evidence of its value in other circumstances.

(2) *Sublingual provocative food testing.* This is based on the claim that there is sufficient absorption of ingested substances through the sublingual mucosa to provoke (like sublingual glyceryl trinitrate in angina) a mild systemic response. It may be used solely as a form of provocative test, or in conjunction with sublingual therapy, which will be further discussed later. The validity of this test is highly doubtful, and a number of recent studies have shown that sublingual provocative food testing does not discriminate between controls and food extracts (Committee on Provocative Food Testing, 1973; Breneman *et al.*, 1974; Lehman, 1980a).

(3) *Intradermal skin testing* as originally described by Rinkel (1949a,b,c). This is discussed later under therapeutic regimes. In the hands of the non-enthusiast the method does not seem to work, and there is considerable doubt as to its efficacy as a diagnostic test for food allergy (Hirsch *et al.*, 1981).

(4) *Cytotoxic food tests in the diagnosis of food allergy.* This type of testing was originally described by Black (1956), who claimed that food allergens will lyse leucocytes of food-allergic patients. The buffy coat from centrifuged venous blood is incubated with the suspected food allergen for a variable period of time (usually about 2 hours), and the number of lysed white cells observed. A recent paper by Lehman (1980b) showed that though this test was reproducible on a single occasion, it fluctuated so extensively from day to day that it was of no diagnostic value.

ORTHODOX AND UNORTHODOX TREATMENT REGIMES

There are three main approaches to the problem of food allergy and intolerance.

(1) Avoidance of the food

It is clearly sensible to avoid foods which—for whatever reason—are a cause of symptoms. However, this is not always easy when patients are intolerant to eggs, milk, or other substances which are commonly used in cooking. Patients on an egg-free or milk-free regime are thus allowed a very limited diet.

This may have encouraged the development of the 'rotating diet', which is much favoured by ecologists. Rinkel *et al.* (1951) suggested that some food sensitizations were transitory: thus, refraining from the ingestion of such foods for a period of days or weeks might permit the food to be eaten once without clinical manifestations. However, frequent ingestion of the food after the period of abstinence might be expected to reinstate the sensitivity. Thus they suggest the use of a rotating diet—and if 'food allergies' are multiple this may be a very complicated process. The scientific basis for such a diet remains unclear.

(2) Anti-allergic drugs

If the patient is shown to be food-allergic rather than food-intolerant, drugs such as disodium cromoglycate may be considered. Their use is discussed in Chapter 6. Where symptoms result from the absorption of the food, rather than from an allergic reaction in the intestine itself, these drugs may be of limited value, however. As most chromones in present use are not absorbed, their possible efficacy is lost.

(3) Hyposensitization regimes

Hyposensitization regimes provide a potentially attractive approach to the problem. Since children tend to outgrow their food allergies (particularly to milk—Kuitunen et al., 1975), it could well be that some sort of natural hyposensitization process occurs, which could be encouraged by appropriate treatment. Hyposensitization regimes are, however, open to a number of criticisms in the way they have been applied to the many patients who are said to have food allergy on vague and inadequate grounds.

Such regimes in the treatment of allergy are still a considerable source of controversy, though they have been in vogue for the past 70 years. Noon (1911) and Freeman (1911) both believed that pollen produced a toxin which caused allergy, and therefore used an immunization technique to produce active immunity. Subsequently Cooke et al. (1935) found that the injection of serum, taken from patients who had been hyposensitized to ragweed, could reduce symptoms in previously untreated patients, and he assumed that hyposensitization had induced the production of blocking antibodies. This hypothesis still has its advocates, but it is now known that hyposensitization cannot be due to this phenomenon alone (Lichtenstein et al., 1968). Hyposensitization regimes have certainly been shown, in controlled studies, to be effective in patients with allergic rhinitis and in some patients with asthma; but the controlled trial technique has not been satisfactorily applied to the treatment of food allergy. The usual reason given for the lack of critical analysis is that it would be wrong to withhold effective treatment even for the short period of a trial, merely in order to see whether the treatment works. The argument will appeal only to those who prefer simple belief rather than an attempt to establish the evidence.

Immunotherapy in the treatment of patients with allergic rhinitis, asthma, and allergy to *Hymenoptera* venoms is now well established. Modern practice involves serial subcutaneous injections of extracts of relevant allergens, administered in progressively increasing doses over a period of months (and usually repeated each year) until a potent immunogenic dose is achieved: this may be monitored by immunological investigations which—to take hay fever as an example—will show (1) an increase in specific serum IgG antibodies to the allergen; (2) an increase in serum IgE antibodies during the first few months, followed by a slow decline in specific IgE over many years; (3) an increase in specific IgG and IgA antibodies in nasal secretions, in the patient who has been successfully treated. The exact mechanisms of such hyposensitization techniques are still not understood. Blocking IgG antibodies may be important but it is interesting to note that, if a crude extract of antigens is used for treatment, antibodies may be demonstrated against those particular antigens even in patients who have not responded to the treatment. It seems likely that the induction of T lymphocyte suppression of the allergic response is also important.

In the case of food allergy, there is little evidence either that 'hypo-sensitization' is effective or that it induces any immunological change. Indeed, the time course which is followed would imply that, if the method is effective at all, it must be through a different mechanism. Frankland (1973) has used 'rush hyposensitization' in highly allergic patients with confirmed food allergy of severe degree, and has sometimes noted a remarkable improvement. Similar observations have been made by B. J. Freedman (personal communication). The method (Freeman, 1930) involves three phases. The patient is hospitalized for phases 1 and 2, a positive prick test to the food having been previously established. Phase 1 comprises large increments of allergen injected subcutaneously at 20-minute intervals to detect the minimal dose to which the patient reacts, and this determines the starting dose for hyposensitization. For instance 0.1 ml of 10^{-9} fish extract is initially injected, followed by 10^{-8}, 10^{-7}, etc., until a local reaction appears. Phase 2 is started at least 3 hours after the phase 1 local reaction. The dose to which the patient reacted is repeated and subsequent injections are given at 3-hour intervals at an increasing dosage, such that a tenfold increase is achieved after a further four injections. The top dose is repeated once a week for 1 month, once a fortnight for the next month and then monthly thereafter (Phase 3). In successful cases, small amounts of food such as egg which has previously provoked anaphy-lactic reactions can be given by mouth within 1 month of starting treatment. In other cases the patient can again take normal quantities of the food involved — a sequence which has been noted for both fish and milk (A. W. Frankland, personal communication). Some patients may, however, be unable to complete the treatment, and measures for dealing with anaphylaxis should be kept to hand.

In the USA low-dose hyposensitization regimes are favoured, based on those described by Rinkel (1949a,b,c) and Miller (1977). In these regimes the food extract is injected intradermally at a concentration which is sufficient to produce a local wealing reaction (and is likely to elicit mild symptoms of the patient's original food allergy, e.g. wheezing or angioedema). Injections are then repeated with ever-increasing dilutions until the 'neutralizing dose' is established, at which dose there is no evidence of a local response after 10 minutes. This is then used as the dosage for regular 'immunotherapy' — higher dilutions being avoided because they increasingly are said to cause severe symptoms of food allergy. Treatment consists of giving the 'neutralizing dose' either sublingually three times daily, or daily subcutaneously. Sublingual therapy is then continued for several years and subcutaneous therapy for variable periods, depending on the physician. Leaving aside arguments about a regime which induces physician-dependence over a period of years and has a doubtful theoretical validity, its clinical efficacy has been challenged by a number of physicians. The efficacy of such a regime — admittedly in allergic rhinitis rather than in food allergy — was tested by the American Academy of

Allergy who sponsored a 2-year double-blind multicentre trial (Hirsch *et al.*, 1981). As reported by Lehman (1980a) double-blind studies have also been carried out in which patients with suspected food allergy were challenged with sublingual food drops or with placebo. No difference could be demonstrated.

Advice from non-medical organizations associated with allergy

To some extent the success of fringe medicine—both in diagnosis and treatment—reflects the failure of the orthodox. Indeed witch doctors, apothecaries, and physicians have all, in turn, failed to satisfy their more critical clients. It is the customer's privilege that he may then turn to alternative systems, which are particularly likely to thrive at times when orthodoxy is most under attack.

At their worst, unorthodox approaches to medicine offer little more than a confidence trick, in which diagnostic services or a dramatically effective treatment is offered for a fee, without any basis or justification for the claims made. At other times a genuine innovation is offered—again, for a fee—with the knowledge that evidence of efficacy is still lacking. Some of the treatments for food allergy which have so far been described fall into this category. The innovator's approach can be justified if he is prepared to evaluate what he does. Often, however, he is not prepared to do this, and critical examination may be undertaken only reluctantly and after an insistence by licensing authorities that his claims are either justified or withdrawn. By this time many patients may have subjected themselves to treatment which is both costly and ineffective.

When the medical profession has been willing to examine the claims of the unorthodox there have, indeed, been benefits—spinal manipulation has been learned from the osteopaths, counter-stimulation techniques from the acupuncturists, and insect-sting immunotherapy from the old-style allergists. Many of the approaches to treatment which have so far been reviewed, although of unproven efficacy, need to be considered in this sympathetic context. However, many unorthodox approaches are less well substantiated and do not fall into this category.

Numerous organizations are concerned with an undefined range of 'allergic' diseases, perhaps emphasizing how many people feel the need for help which is not provided by the medical profession. Their existence is no guarantee of their quality. Many of these are based in the United Kingdom, but a number of corresponding organizations are present in other countries. One advisory service claims to identify patients' allergies from a sample of their hair using Radionic equipment. This service costs between £6 and £10 and for this the patient receives a list of foods and other chemicals to which the 'analysis' of their hair suggests they are allergic, together with some general advice on avoidance diets in the treatment of food allergies. This organization is also prepared to analyse hair to define whether the patient suffers from vitamin and mineral deficiencies, which costs a further £6. Based on this testing a 'mega-vitamin' diet may be recommended or the avoidance of aluminium and lead cooking vessels. They also suggest that the patient's hair should be re-analysed after 6 months. Our only experience of this organization was when one of us (R. St.C.B.) sent hair from a patient who had an excellent history of angioedema following the ingestion of eggs and fish, and who had positive skin prick tests and radio-allergosorbent tests to both allergens. Testing of this patient's hair apparently showed him to be 'allergic to cow's milk and cheese' and he was advised to avoid both. The patient was also offered details of the 'pulse test' and auto-immune urine therapy for a further fee.

A second organization which has an interest in food allergy, and is prepared to give advice on the subject, is the 'Radionic Association', which has functioned in the UK for over 6 years and offers advice on treating both humans and animals. There is a school of radionics which trains students to use radionic equipment and to interpret the results. All that is required is a snippet of the patient's hair (called a 'witness') which acts as a link between the Radionics treatment ('which measures electromagnetic radiations of various frequencies') and the patient wherever he may be. The main work of this organization in humans involves patients with symptoms of inhalant and food allergy, schizophrenia, depression, and other illnesses affecting the brain and central nervous system, and those with epilepsy and migraine. After testing, the patient is recommended to eliminate the food which has been found to be causing 'allergic' symptoms.

The initiator of Radionics was a San Francisco physician, Dr Abrams, who early in the twentieth century percussed a patient's abdomen in the erect position and found that areas of dullness and hollowness appear to vary with the points of the compass. He then went on to develop this observation and noted considerable variation in the 'electromagnetic radiation patterns' emitted from different individuals if they were ill. The findings were then extrapolated to the diagnosis and treatment of the disease, neither of which requires the patient's presence. For the interested reader, several accounts of the 'science' of Radionics are available. Probably the most comprehensive work is the book *Report on Radionics* by Edward Russell (1973).

A further organization exists which is willing to give advice on food allergy together with a long list of books, including those on the subject of ecology, allergy in general, the use of dieting in cancer, and autoimmune urine therapy. The dangers which are inherent in an uncritical dietary approach are seen in the case of a patient with operable carcinoma of the breast, who has been attending the Breast Clinic in Edinburgh but refused surgery because she had first read an article entitled 'Cancer therapy by the Gentler Method', i.e. by food elimination. In the meantime her carcinoma has spread and has become inoperable. While it might be reasonable to suggest diets for patients with irreversible diseases such as multiple sclerosis, where they are unlikely to cause harm, the same is clearly not true of early malignant disease, where conventional treatment may be wholly effective provided it is instituted without delay.

The recommendation of autoimmune urine therapy deserved more detailed consideration. Indeed, the magical properties of urine have a long history, and the ingestion of urine as a cure for disease has been practised all over the world for several centuries. India's former Prime Minister, Mr Desai, drank his own urine daily and used to alarm diplomats visiting his residence when he offered them a drink, because they always wondered what ingredients were included! Their fears may have been misplaced, according to a book on the subject recommended by the same organization called *The Water of Life, a Treatise on Urine Therapy*. This book, by John Armstrong (1971), was originally published in 1944. It includes a number of case histories, describing patients with various diseases who had ingested urine — usually their own — with some ameliorative effect. A much more disturbing booklet is that entitled *The Use of Injected and Sublingual Urine in the Treatment of Allergies — a Preliminary Report* by Dr A. P. Dunne. This seeks to rationalize autoimmune urine therapy, in which patients inject themselves or their children with their own urine. The author claims (without evidence) that antibodies to allergens have been observed 'to accurately reconstruct themselves into functioning immuno-globulins in the urine'. The contention is that these antibodies might be useful in the treatment of allergic disease. Explicit instructions are given as to filtration of the urine, and doses are injected subcutaneously into the buttock, according to the body weight of the subject. Patients who are over 200 lb in weight inject themselves with 8 ml (!); infants are given 2 ml. Injections are repeated weekly until the patient becomes asymptomatic — which may, according to the author, take 3–4 months. Treatment may also be effected by sublingual administration.

The pseudo-scientific approach is not without danger. While it would be arrogant for doctors to think that all fringe medicine is therapy by lunatics for lunatics, some critical examination is essential in order to avoid misleading the public and — even more so — some of the more gullible and sensation-seeking publicists of press and television. The fact that no scientific explanation is available at present does not alter the fact that some of the unorthodox phenomena described in books on subjects such as food allergy may well have some scientific basis. It is necessary, however, to outline some of the unacceptable facets of fringe medicine, so that the patient is not positively harmed. This has been the chief object of this section.

The warning about 'pseudoscientific' organizations should perhaps be extended to three particular groups of individuals for whom conventional medicine has failed:

(1) those with 'no-hope' diseases, which cause prolonged disability in spite of medical efforts—diseases such as multiple sclerosis and rheumatoid arthritis, or even fatal diseases such as cancer;
(2) parents of children with distressing diseases such as severe atopic eczema;
(3) neurotics and those with other psychiatric disorders who are prone to clutch at straws, and who turn to 'food allergy' merely as one of the most recently publicized explanations for their ills.

In many cases, with neither a soundly based diagnosis nor a clear rationale, patients have been encouraged to go to endless lengths to avoid certain foods. They may also be asked to follow regimes which require obsessional observance and to undertake prolonged 'cures' which continue for months or years. The main hazards result not from modest dieting (provided that the nutritional aspects are considered) but from the false hopes which may be engendered and from the variety of bizarre treatments which may be recommended—and given—to the patient's detriment.

REFERENCES

Andresen, A. F. R. (1942). Ulcerative colitis—allergic phenomenon. *American Journal of Digestive Diseases*, **9**, 91.
Armstrong, J. (1971). *The Water of Life. A Treatise on Urine Therapy* (2nd edition). Health Science Press, Devon.
Baker, R. W. R., Thompson, R. H. S., and Zilkha, K. J. (1964). Serum fatty acids in multiple sclerosis. *Journal of Neurology, Neurosurgery and Psychiatry*, **27**, 408.
Barnetson, R. St. C., Merrett, T. G., and Ferguson, A. (1981). Studies on hypo-immunoglobulin E in atopic diseases with particular reference to food allergens. *Clinical and Experimental Immunology*, **46**, 54.
Bates, D., Fawcett, P. R. W., Shaw, D. A., and Weightman, D. (1978). Poly-unsaturated fatty acids in treatment of acute remitting multiple sclerosis. *British Medical Journal*, **4**, 1390.
Black, A. P. (1956). A new diagnostic method in allergic disease. *Pediatrics*, **17**, 716.
Braathen, L. R., Baklien, K., Horig, T., Fausa, O. and Brandtzaeg, P. (1980). Immunological, histological and electron-microscopical investigations of the gut in atopic dermatitis. *Acta Dermatovenereologica*, Suppl. 92, 78.
Breneman, J. C., Hurst, A., Heiner, D., Leney, F. L., Morris, D. and Josephson, B. M. (1974). Final report of the Food Allergy Committee of the American College of Allergists on the clinical evaluation of sublingual provocative testing method for diagnosis of food allergy. *Annals of Allergy*, **33**, 164.
Brown, M., Gibney, M., Husband, P. R., and Radcliffe, M. (1981). Food allergy in polysymptomatic patients. *Practitioner*, **225**, 1651.
Cam, C. and Nigogosyan, G. (1963). Acquired toxic porphyria cutanea tarda due to hexachlorobenzene. *Journal of the American Medical Association*, **183**, 88.
Coca, A. F. (1942). *Familial non-reaginic food allergy*, Charles C. Thomas, Springfield, Illinois and Blackwell Scientific Publications, Oxford.
Committee on Provocative Food Testing (1973). *Annals of Allergy*, **31**, 375.
Cooke, R. A., Barnard, J. H., Hebald, S., and Stull, A. (1935). Serological evidence of immunity with coexisting sensitisation in type of human allergy (hay fever). *Journal of Experimental Medicine*, **62**, 733.

Coombs, R. R. A., and Gell, P. G. H. (1963). In *Clinical Aspects of Immunology* (eds P. G. H. Gell and R. R. A. Coombs). Blackwell, Oxford.

Dickey, L. D. (1976). *Clinical Ecology*. Charles C. Thomas, Springfield, Illinois.

Doherty, M., and Barry, R. E. (1981). Gluten-induced mucosal changes in subjects without overt small bowel disease. *Lancet*, **1**, 517.

Dong, C. H., and Banks, J. (1976). *New Hope for the Arthritic*. Hart-Davis, MacGibbon, London.

Frankland, A. W. (1973). Allergy: immunity gone wrong. *Proceedings of the Royal Society of Medicine*, **66**, 365.

Freeman, J. (1911). Further observations on the treatment of hay fever by hypodermic inoculation of pollen vaccine. *Lancet*, **2**, 814.

Freeman, J. (1930). 'Rush' inoculation, with special reference to hay fever treatment. *Lancet*, **1**, 744.

Harrington, J. M., and Waldron, H. A. (1981). The effects of work exposures on organ systems. I—Liver, kidney and bladder. In: *Occupational Health Practice* (ed. R. J. F. Schilling), 2nd edition. Butterworths, London, pp.89–114.

Hench, P. S., and Rosenberg, E. F. (1941). Palindromic rheumatism. A 'new' oft-recurring disease of joints apparently producing no articular residues: report of 34 cases. *Proceedings of the Staff Meetings of the Mayo Clinic*, **16**, 808.

Hirsch, S. R., Kalbfleisch, J. H., Golbert, T. M., Josephson, B. M., McConnell, L. H., Scanlon, R., Kniker, W. T., Fink, J. N., Murphree, J. J., and Cohen, S. H. (1981). Rinkel injection therapy: a multicentre controlled study. *Journal of Allergy and Clinical Immunology*, **68**, 133.

Hunter, D. (1978). *The Diseases of Occupation*, 6th edition. Hodder and Stoughton, London.

Jewell, D. P., and Truelover, S. C. (1972). Circulating antibodies to cow's milk protein in ulcerative colitis. *Gut*, **13**, 796.

King, D. S. (1981). Can allergic exposure provoke psychological symptoms? A double-blind test. *Biological Psychiatry*, **16**, 3.

Kuitunen, P., Visakorpi, J. K., Savilahti, E., and Pelkoven, P. (1975). Malabsorption syndrome with cow's milk intolerance. Clinical findings and course in 54 cases. *Archives of Diseases of Children*, **50**, 351.

Lancet (1982). Editorial. Food additives and hyperactivity. *Lancet*, **1**, 662.

Lehman, C. W. (1980a). A double-blind study of sublingual provocative food testing: a study of its efficacy. *Annals of Allergy*, **45**, 144.

Lehman, C. W. (1980b). The leukocytic food allergy test: a study of its reliability and reproducibility. Effect of diet and sublingual food drops on this test. *Annals of Allergy*, **45**, 150.

Lessof, M. H., Wraith, D. G., Merrett, T. G., Merrett, J., and Buisseret, P. D. (1980). Food allergy and intolerance in 100 patients—local and systemic effects. *Quarterly Journal of Medicine*, **195**, 259.

Lichenstein, L. M., Norman, P. S., and Winkenwerder, W. L. (1968). Clinical and *in vitro* studies on the role of immunotherapy in ragweed hay fever. *American Journal of Medicine*, **44**, 514.

Mackarness, R. (1976). *Not All In The Mind*. Pan Books, London.

Mackarness, R. (1980). *Chemical Victims*. Pan Books, London.

Millar, J. H. D., Zilkha, K. J., Langman, M. J. S., Payling Wright, H., Smith, A. D., Belin, J., and Thompson, R. H. S. (1973). Double-blind trial of linoleate supplementation of the diet in multiple sclerosis. *British Medical Journal*, **1**, 765.

Miller, J. B. (1977). A double-blind study of food extract injection therapy: a preliminary report. *Annals of Allergy*, **38**, 185.

Nixon, P. G. F. (1982). 'Total allergy syndrome' or fluctuating hypocarbia? *Lancet*, **1**, 516.

Noon, L. (1911). Prophylactic inoculation against hay fever. *Lancet*, **1**, 1572.

O'Morain, C., Segal, A. W., and Levi, A. J. (1980). Elemental diets in treatment of acute Crohn's disease. *British Medical Journal*, **4**, 1173.

O'Shea, J. A., and Porter, S. F. (1981). Double-blind study of children with hyperkinetic syndrome treated with multi-allergen extract sublingually. *J. Learning Disabilities*, **14**, 189–191.

Paganelli, R., Levinsky, R. J., Brostoff, J. and Wraith, D. G. (1979). Immune complexes containing food proteins in normal and atopic subjects after oral challenge and effect of sodium cromoglycate on antigen absorption. *Lancet*, **1**, 1270–1272.

Parke, A., and Hughes, G. R. V. (1981). Rheumatoid arthritis and food: a case study. *British Medical Journal*, **2**, 2027.

Pirquet, C. von (1906). Allergie. *Münchner Medizinische Wochenschrift*, **53**, 1457.

Rapp, D. R. (1978). Does diet affect hyperactivity? *Journal of Learning Disabilities*, **11**, 56.

Rapp, D. R. (1979). Food allergy treatment for hyperkinesis. *Journal of Learning Disabilities*, **12**, 42.

Rinkel, H. J. (1944). The role of food allergy in internal medicine. *Annals of Allergy*, **2**, 115.

Rinkel, H. J., Randolph, T. G. Y., and Zeller, M. (1951). *Food Allergy*. Charles C. Thomas, Springfield, Illinois.

Rinkel, H. J. (1949a). Inhalant allergy. I. The whealing response of the skin to serial dilution testing. *Annals of Allergy*, **7**, 625.

Rinkel, H. J. (1949b). Inhalant allergy. II. Factors modifying the whealing response of the skin. *Annals of Allergy*, **7**, 631.

Rinkel, H. J. (1949c). Inhalant allergy. III. The co-seasonal application of serial dilution testing (titration). *Annals of Allergy*, **7**, 639.

Rowe, A. H. (1931). *Food Allergy: its manifestations and diagnosis and treatment, with a general discussion of bronchial asthma*. Lee & Febiger, Philadelphia.

Russell, E. (1973). *Report on Radionics*. Neville Spearman, Sudbury.

Shatin, R. (1964). Multiple sclerosis and geography. New interpretation of epidemiological observations. *Neurology (Minneapolis)*, **13**, 338.

Sköldstam, L., Larsson, L., and Lindström, F. D. (1979). Effects of fasting and lactovegetarian diet on rheumatoid arthritis. *Scandinavian Journal of Rheumatology*, **8**, 249.

Solis-Cohen, S. (1914). On some angioneural arthroses (periarthroses, pararthroses) commonly mistaken for gout or rheumatism. *American Journal of Medical Sciences*, **147**, 228.

Swank, R. L. (1950). Multiple sclerosis; correlation of its incidence with dietary fat. *American Journal of Medical Sciences*, **220**, 421.

Tabuenca, J. M. (1981). Toxic–allergic syndrome caused by ingestion of rapeseed oil denatured with aniline. *Lancet*, **2**, 567.

Tichy, J., Vymagal, J., and Michalec, C. (1969). Serum lipoproteins, cholesterol esters and phospholipids in multiple sclerosis. *Acta Neurologica Scandinavica*, **45**, 32.

Truelove, S. C. (1961). Ulcerative colitis provoked by milk. *British Medical Journal*, **1**, 154.

Vaughan, W. T. (1943). Palindromic rheumatism among allergic persons. *Journal of Allergy*, **14**, 256.

Wraith, D. G. (1980). Clinical manifestations. In: *The First Food Allergy Workshop* (ed. R. R. A. Coombs), pp.42–3.

Wright, R., Morton, J. A., and Taylor, K. B. (1965). Immunological studies in multiple sclerosis: incidence of circulating antibodies to dietary proteins and auto-antigens. *British Medical Journal*, **1**, 491.

Clinical Reactions to Food
Edited by M. H. Lessof
© 1983 J. Hubert Lacey. Published 1983 John Wiley & Sons Ltd.

The Patient's Attitude to Food

J. Hubert Lacey

Academic Department of Psychiatry,
St George's Hospital Medical School, London

It is self-evident that food is necessary for survival. However, the processes of social and emotional development have forged complex and highly variable attitudes towards both food and the act of eating. Some attitudes stem directly from the nutrient function of food. Thus the growth, preparation, serving, and eating of food has a central place in all societies, even when human survival is not threatened by scarcity or famine. However, other attitudes are more distant. Thus, in women especially, the relationship between food, shape, and weight can lead to shame and guilt, in part because of the association with sexuality. Food is a vital element in the relationship between mother and child: it is seen as an expression of love. The mechanism has been more generally applied, and emotions which are superficially unrelated to nutrition have nevertheless been invested in food. These emotions and mechanisms, both in their general incidence and pathology, are the subject matter of this chapter.

NORMAL ATTITUDES TO FOOD

If eating is the final common pathway for a wealth of emotional and biological needs, it is not surprising that there should be wide variation in energy and nutritional intake between individuals and within the same individual at different times. This has been shown for children (DHSS, 1975) and for adults (Widdowson and McCance, 1936; Thomson, 1958), variation being most marked amongst adolescents (Huenemann and Turner, 1942; Yudkin, 1951) — perhaps because of rapid growth and immature emotions.

Marked variation in energy and carbohydrate intake was shown in a recent study of the eating habits of 16–17-year-old schoolgirls (Lacey *et al.*, 1978). The study demonstrated that eating behaviour previously considered to be unusual or abnormal was widespread. The girls demonstrated two distinct patterns of energy intake, each with its own periodicity. The first cycle was short and varied markedly day by day, with a tendency for the girls to eat more during the weekend. The mean daily variation of calorific intake amongst the girls was fourfold. These daily swings were superimposed on a further cycle with a periodicity of about a month, energy intake tending to increase prior to menstruation and to decline immediately after it. This energy fluctuation was, in the main, secondary to carbohydrate manipulation. Protein and fat intake tended to remain more stable.

The study showed that periods of carbohydrate abstention or avoidance were closely followed by a period of eating in which mainly carbohydrate foods were sought. Whilst this was a feature exhibited by most of the girls, in some the pattern was more dramatic, and their eating had a 'bingeing' quality (bulimia). The reason for this must be contentious, but the sustained insulin response that follows initial ingestion of carbohydrate may itself promote continued carbohydrate ingestion and lead to the craving for carbohydrates which mark these 'bingeing' periods (Crisp, 1981).

Faddism, mild bulimia and 'dieting' are usually inseparable and, in their less intense form, ubiquitous in young female populations.

A study examining the total teenage population of a small Swedish town (Nylander, 1971) revealed that many girls thought themselves fat, and this feeling became common with increasing adolescent age, being reported by only 26 per cent of the 14-year-olds but by over half of the 18-year-olds in the sample. Only 7 per cent of 18-year-old boys thought themselves to be fat. A further study looked at approximately 1000 teenagers in the American Public High School system (Huenemann et al., 1966). The results revealed that teenagers have a great interest in body configuration. The girls were particularly preoccupied with their shape and weight: about 50 per cent of the girls classified themselves as obese, whereas only 25 per cent of them were identified as such in anthropometric terms.

In the Swedish study, about one-third of the girls reported serious dietary manipulation. This, too, was age-related, being more frequent amongst the older teenage girls (76 per cent of 17-year-olds) and, not surprisingly, amongst those whose weight was above average. For the majority of girls 'dieting' was fairly ineffectual, in that only small body-weight losses were reported. However, a substantial proportion of all girls reported that they had developed symptoms which were connected with their dietary manipulation. Thus, 10 per cent of the sample described amenorrhoea and increased interest in food and food preparation within the context of 'dieting', faddism, or compulsive over-eating. The number of girls who reported major weight losses increased with age.

More recently, Crisp (1981) reported that in his study of schoolgirls the majority were concerned about their weight and were attempting to lose it by dieting. Concern increased as they passed through menarche (27 per cent of pre-menarchal girls were concerned about their weight compared with 48 per cent of those who were post-menarchal). Crisp also reported frequent vomiting in 3·2 per cent of his population, and that this symptom was related to concern about being too 'fat'. From Canada it has been reported that in a middle-class suburban population 5 per cent of women vomited periodically as a means of controlling body weight (Cleghorn and Brown, 1964).

'Dieting' is pervasive amongst young women. The behaviour seems to be associated with the perception these young girls have of their bodies and the sociocultural factors which have influenced them. Since World War II the desired female shape has become more angular and lean. Orbach (1978) has claimed this to be a function of a male-orientated society. However, there is little evidence that men prefer any particular shape in women and certainly not that excessive thinness is held as desirable. Rather society, as a whole, seems to hold in esteem an 'ideal' which has fluctuated through the ages. The shape and weight of ballet dancers provides a good example of how feminine beauty has varied to reflect the aesthetic standards of a particular epoch: the ballet dancers of Degas are very different from those of a modern troupe. Similarly, the Hollywood actresses of the 1930s differ markedly from Twiggy. This recent shift towards thinness was demonstrated by Garner *et al.* (1980) who showed that the *Playboy* centrefold models and the 'Miss America Pageant' contestants showed a trend towards being taller, having larger waists, and smaller hips and bust. Interestingly, the same overall movement to thinness has occurred in the shape of consumer durables: the modern angular Metro is very different from the curved, plump Morris Minor. Having said this, it is reasonable to add that women in our society are expected to be more responsive to fashion than are men, and, as we know that in those subcultures in which there is excessive pressure to slim (models, ballet dancers) there is a greater incidence of eating disorders, it follows that society's pressure will lead women, as a whole, to be more susceptible to dieting, faddism, and bulimia.

In more general populations, over-perception of body shape, previously thought to be a hallmark of anorexia nervosa, is now found to be common amongst all late teenage girls. The degree of over-perception is less than amongst anorectics, but still substantial. Thighs are particularly over-perceived, and the erroneous body shape generally held is reminiscent of the exaggerated female form of a fertility goddess—a collective unconscious indeed! Unlike boys, who see their bodies as a whole (Crisp and Kalucy, 1974) and exercise to 'keep fit', girls tend to perceive their bodies part by part and attempt to deal—by dieting—with any area which gives them dissatisfaction. This tendency for late adolescent girls to over-perceive their body shape has implications for their attitude to food and the pervasiveness of 'dieting'.

Thus, dietary restriction, mild bulimia, over-estimation of body shape, and undue preoccupation with body weight, are widespread features in young female populations and are not uncommon in more general populations.

FADDISM

Food likes and dislikes are common. The physician's advice is rarely sought, except when the behaviour disorder is severe. Fads are particularly common in the infant, the adolescent, and in those under stress.

Food refusal in infancy is usually part of a more general negativism. The infant may refuse certain kinds of food, or refuse lumpy food, or wish to regress to baby foods or a bottle, or to being fed by his mother. Later feeding problems can be laid down during this time, as parents battle and cajole their infant: the conflict lying between the need of parents to be sure their child is properly fed and the drive of the infant for increasing autonomy (Berry Brazelton, 1976). The conflict is heightened because food is an expression of love a mother has for her child, and food refusal appears to both recipient and donor as love rejected.

As the infant becomes a child, a particular food can be invested with emotion and be used, with the mother's sanction, to console and comfort. Faddism can become more pathological when love is given less as an intangible and more in the substantial form of food. The 'fad' is not only special to the child but also to the mother, and it symbolizes, in a pathological way, the specialness of the relationship between them. When faddism develops to this degree it tends to become generalized, infecting a range of foods, which have a tendency to be either sweet or starchy. Changes in the child's emotional state tend to lead to him being given food. Normal responses to affective change are not learned: sadness is not appreciated, nor discomfort acted upon — except by the passive response of eating. An unsurprising result is childhood obesity, which in some families is valued as evidence of good mothering or good health. The child's shape is thus a reflection of his mother's anxiety, insecurity, or neurotic propensity. The end result is to confuse, in the child's mind, the subtle reinforcing experiences concerned with the relationship between hunger and satiety on the one hand and his own developing autonomy on the other (Kalucy, 1976).

Adolescence is a time when the personality traits fuse to form the character of the adult. It is a time of exploration and enquiry, and it would be silly to deny that food likes and dislikes are not a part of normal experimentation. However, such benign and normal behaviour can become a malignant pivot of neurotic activity. The fear of approaching independence from parents, or anger and resentment of dependence on them, especially if heightened by sexual unsureness, may exacerbate previously learned childhood habits (although, in late adolescence and early adulthood the role of the patient is less crucial and interpersonal relationships more important).

Neurotic faddism is a changeable caprice which varies on presentation from a whim to a freakish craze. It tends to revolve around the active search for particular carbohydrate foods. The food is chosen superficially for its availability, sweetness, or the sense of fulness it brings. More deeply, and usually unconsciously, the 'choice' reflects the symbolism of the particular food, learned from infancy. Alternatively, it is possible that the tendency to fixate on carbohydrates may be related to its evolutionary importance in maintaining fat deposits, whose procreative importance will be alluded to later.

Fads may also develop as a response to real or imagined allergic reactions. The desired or avoided food is thus a single food or conceptual series of foods, not a biologically similar class of food. The author has noted how, under neurotic parental pressure and medical zeal, such faddism can become so extensive that a 'total' or near-total 'allergy syndrome' develops. This has not been the subject of psychological study but the cases treated by the author presented clinically as secondary anorexia nervosa of an abstaining type. What marks out such patients from the true anorectic is first, a lack of a phobia of normal weight (see below)—the patient welcomes returning to a normal weight with none of the associated emotional turmoil of the primary anorectic. Second, there is a positive family history of food allergy or asthma which sensitizes the family to the 'danger' of food and is interpreted by the patient psychologically. Further the parents, whilst intelligent, seem to be remarkably gullible, and their preoccupation with food reached its height during the patient's early adolescence. The patients give the impression of being 'passive pawns in a game being played by their parents'.

ABNORMAL ATTITUDES TO FOOD

The line between what is a normal attitude to food and what is abnormal is not clear-cut. Thus, for example, the degree of over-eating which is necessary to cause distress varies widely and depends more on individual response than the amount of food consumed. Like any neurotic behaviour the severity of a symptom of disordered eating can be construed as a mark on a scale. The scale is individual to each and every one of us, being derived from our genetic and environmental background. The mark will vary in response to stress, especially stress of an interpersonal nature. Symptoms such as substantial weight fluctuation, bulimia, or psychogenic vomiting may form the major feature of the mental state, the patient displacing her emotions on them, thereby forming one of the eating disorders. Alternatively, such symptoms may be associated with any neurotic or psychotic disorder and, although disturbing, are not central to the clinical presentation. This will be dealt with later under 'Food and other mood states'.

The eating disorders are usually divided into three categories: massive obesity, the bulimic syndrome, and anorexia nervosa. However, it would be misleading to imagine that patients are diagnosed according to their presenting weight: the diagnosis of anorexia nervosa for instance must be made on psychological grounds (at times, the body weight of an anorectic—particularly a bulimic anorectic—can reach near-normal levels). Similarly, with strenuous effort, the massively obese can lose substantial amounts of fat, yet the psychopathology remains. That having been said, it would be misleading again to deny the close interrelationship of the three conditions. Thus, the bulimic syndrome can best be judged as a sub-group of obesity—massive obesity being thwarted by vomiting-back the excess food ingested. Further, anorectics, after intensive re-feeding in hospital, can develop a post-anorectic syndrome which superficially is very similar to the bulimic syndrome (although, of course, the pathognomonic psychological features of anorexia nervosa remain).

The most noteworthy aspect of all the eating disorders is that the complainants are overwhelmingly women. An attempt to understand these disorders must focus on this observation and attempt to explain it. The very fact that there is such a profound discrepancy between the sexes in their attitudes to food suggests that the pathology is rooted in sexuality. This is not to imply that the problem is one of sexual dysfunction (and associated, therefore, with the act of intercourse), but rather that it is related to those concepts which differentiate masculinity and femininity, both biologically and socially.

Superficially, what marks out an adult woman from a man is her size and shape—the differences in shape being composed, in the main, of fat tissue. Women are more fatty than men—a healthy woman having twice as much body fat as a man, whereas a man has one and a half times the lean body mass and one and a half times the skeletal mass of a woman (Brook, 1981).

This relationship between fat and female sexuality is emphasized by the timing in a woman's life when fat is deposited, the sites of those deposits and their function.

The first rapid increase in fat deposition occurs at puberty. Further fat deposition occurs during pregnancy and sometimes at the menopause, events which are sexually determined. In the pubescent girl, first sexual emotions are associated with, and emphasized by, a dramatic change in shape and weight, and by menstruation. These events declare to the girl, her family, and her peers that she is preparing, psychologically and physiologically, for reproduction. They draw attention to the changing nature of relationships both within and without the family, and for the need for new social skills about which she feels unsure.

The profound changes in female body shape are the result of a general increase in subcutaneous fat, together with concentrations of fat tissues at specific sites, especially the thighs, the breasts, and the buttocks. Gluteal fat deposits are further emphasized in pubescence as the bony pelvis grows and the transverse diameter increases. Such deposits tend to delineate the female from the male, and hence have developed secondary sexual significance.

The fact—that women are fattier than men—begs a question. Why? Any answer is likely to remain contentious. Fat is mostly used in the body as a storage tissue of high energy. Could it be that such fat deposits in women provide, in evolutionary terms, a reserve of sufficient energy to maintain pregnancy and lactation in the face of erratic food supplies? This view is reinforced by the findings that fat tissue mass and body weight appear to act as triggers for the pubertal process itself.

Two threshold weights have, so far, been delineated. Luteinizing hormone (LH) and follicle stimulating hormone (FSH) appear to be unresponsive to their releasing factors below a body weight of 43 kg. Work with an anorexia nervosa population, and with re-feeding in hospital, suggests that a mean body weight of 43 kg is necessary to trigger sexual hormone activity with its attendant feminization and psychological sexuality (Palmer *et al.*, 1975).

A somewhat higher body weight threshold has been suggested for menstruation, although this is more contentious. Rose Frisch, examining a general population of adolescent girls, has determined that menstruation occurs at a mean weight of 48 kg, and when at least 17 per cent of body weight is in the form of fat tissue (Frisch and McArthur, 1974). These two distinct weight thresholds seem to initiate and complete the hormonal process of changing a girl into a woman. Body weight and fat tissue provide the driving force for this biological and psychological change. Given this, it is not perhaps surprising that within the turmoil of pubertal change, dieting and bulimia are widespread amongst teenage school girls because, consciously or unconsciously or unconsciously, the association of their new uncertainty and weight is recognized.

THE EATING DISORDERS

These will be examined as three main disorders.

ANOREXIA NERVOSA

Perhaps it is within anorexia nervosa that the most malignant attitude to food is found. Strictly, anorectics do not have a disordered appetite, nor is food the main focus of their preoccupation. Rather, the disorder centres around body weight. Initially, this is described as a dislike of obesity and a desire to avoid it. Later, and more accurately, they express an intense fear of regaining or re-approaching their *normal* body weight. Whilst most clinicians would agree with Thoma (1967) when he said that the 'most obvious hallmark of anorexia is a physically determined refusal of food', it is this fear of normal adolescent body weight (Crisp, 1967a) which is pathognomonic of the condition and the psychological basis of diagnosis.

Russell (1970) describes this attitude as 'a morbid fear of becoming fat' and uses it as one of his three specific diagnostic criteria. The other criteria are:

(1) an abnormal behaviour consisting of an avoidance of 'fattening' foods, or self-induced vomiting, or purgation, or excessive exercise, which, singularly or in combination, leads to a marked loss of weight;

(2) an endocrine disorder manifest as amenorrhoea in women, or loss of libido in men.

Initially, Russell hypothesized that the endocrine disorder was primary, but now most clinicians feel that the abnormal attitude to weight is at the root of the condition, either with (Crisp, 1977) or without (Bruch, 1965) psychosocial overlay. Some clinicians (Dally, 1969; Feighner *et al.*, 1972) superimpose on this necessary criterion certain quantitative factors. Thus, Feighner states that any anorectic must demonstrate the following features:

(1) age of onset before 25 years;

(2) anorexia with accompanying weight loss of at least 25 per cent of original body weight;

(3) a distorted–implacable attitude towards eating, food or weight that overrides hunger, admonitions, and threats;

(4) no known medical or other psychiatric illness which could account for the anorexia and weight loss;

(5) at least two of the following:
   (a) amenorrhoea,
   (b) lanugo hair,
   (c) bradycardia,
   (d) periods of over-activity,
   (e) bulimia,
   (f) vomiting.

Although the condition may not become manifest until the late teens or twenties, the seeds of the disorder go back to early adolescence. Female pubertal change involves a change in shape composed, in the main, of fat tissue which draws the attention of the male and, more importantly, is associated in the mind of the girl with her own sexuality and impulsivity.

   The future anorectic tends to be pre-morbidly over-weight, and thus reaches earlier those weight thresholds which, as described earlier, act as triggers for the pubertal process. The patient will thus describe having entered the changes of adolescence earlier than her schoolgirl friends who, because they themselves remain pre-pubertal, would not have provided the usual peer support. If, in addition, adolescent unsureness and difficulties associated with adulthood are not discussed at home, the girl may feel very isolated. Being surrounded by the 'dieting' mythology at school, and excessive sensitivity to shape and weight at home, the mildly overweight future anorectic begins to 'diet' seriously (Figure 1). She soon plummets below the 43 kg weight threshold and becomes,

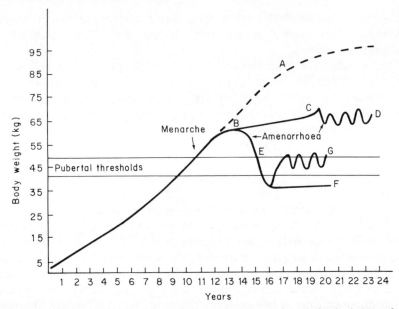

FIGURE 1   *The bulimic patient's progress.* Note: The 'natural destiny' (A) of the bulimic patient is thwarted by social and sexual awareness which leads to dietary restraint (B). An emotional 'crisis' with profound self-doubt triggers a transient weight increase (C) and bulimia and psychogenic vomiting at 'normal' body weight—the bulimic syndrome—follows (D). Massive dieting (E) leads to a weight loss below pubertal thresholds (see text). The carbohydrate-abstaining anorectic (F) remains sexually quiescent whilst the bulimic phase of anorexia nervosa represents a doomed attempt to 'resolve' the anorexia, sexuality being, in part, rekindled (G).

with unconscious relief, sexually quiescent. Of course, she soon realizes that she has 'overdone it' and attempts to regain some weight. However, every time her weight goes above 43 kg sexuality is re-kindled and, with it, all her fears and unsureness. She thus remains biologically and psychologically trapped below 43 kg: a phobia of normal body weight.

The most prominent feature of the anorectic's family is the sense of guilt felt and declared by the parents; yet manifest psychopathology is rare. Within the family there is often someone who is particularly thin or obese, and the significance to the patient of this individual often needs to be pursued. 'Dieting' and concern about weight is common, although it need not be for cosmetic reasons—cardiac problems or diabetes in the family may have led to an altered life-style. Such a change is particularly relevant if it occurs at about the time of the patient's menarche. The families often have a connection with food (farmers, nutritionists, etc.); art and design (ballet, interior design); or health.

Anorexia nervosa can be divided into two groups clinically. The most common group are those anorectics who maintain their low body weight by avoidance of carbohydrate, whilst about 30 per cent of the clinic population (Nemiah, 1958) remain within their weight limits by purgation and psychogenic vomiting.

The carbohydrate abstainers are younger and lighter than the bulimics (see Figure 1). Clinically, they appear emaciated, being usually below 43 kg, and they are amenorrhoeic. Characteristically, they have a fine lanugo hair over their bodies, which presumably develops as a means of heat conservation as their fat insulation is depleted. They are hyperactive and occasionally frenetic. Below 43 kg they have a reversed temperature rhythm which rights itself on weight gain. They claim not to get colds and virus infections, which may be due either to an altered immune response (Armstrong-Esther et al., 1978), or to social isolation. At low body weight they describe a sleep disturbance marked by early-morning waking, although, unlike the depressed, they rarely complain of it. In a study examining anorectics re-feeding in hospital (Lacey et al., 1975), initial weight gain was associated with an increase in slow wave sleep (SWS) which tended to decrease as the weight was finally restored to the mean level of a matched population. It has been suggested that SWS is associated with general bodily synthetic processes, and such processes characterized these patients at this stage of treatment. As target weight approaches there is a dramatic increase in REM (dream) sleep to normal levels. This stage of sleep, which may perhaps be associated with cerebral synthetic activity, occurred during a period of psychotherapy and restoration of reproductive physiology and presumably, therefore, a related increase in cerebral activity.

The abstaining anorectic has a 'pre-pubertal' hormone pattern (Russell and Beardwood, 1968) and is sexually quiescent. She has high ethical standards and is distressed when she is forced by her phobia to lie to her parents and teachers about her food intake. The patient's characteristic emotional immaturity is mirrored by an 'immature' carpal radiograph. The patient's radiological age bears no statistical relationship to her chronological age but is arrested at the age of onset of anorexia and can be calculated as the sum of that age, plus any periods of re-feeding (Lacey et al., 1979).

The bulimic anorectic presents a slightly different clinical picture. She is heavier, being usually about 48 kg, and presents to the clinic at a slightly older age. She often gives a history of being unable to maintain her anorexia by carbohydrate avoidance and most authorities see bulimic anorexia as a malignant extension of the more characteristic avoidance pattern. Because she is heavier, and above the 43 kg threshold of sexual awareness, the bulimic anorectic tends to have sexual feelings (see Figure 1) but is terrified of them. Characteristically, there may be quite marked swings of body weight. Lanugo hair is rare. Teeth, particularly the palatal surfaces, may be eroded from persistent vomiting (Hurst et al., 1977). The patient appears more disturbed psychologically, and the prognosis seems poorer (Crisp, 1977; Crisp et al., 1980b).

The anorectic's fear of food is such that she will insist on preparing her own food and eating alone. She often takes on responsibility for preparing the family's meals and enjoys vicariously over-feeding other family members, particularly younger siblings. It has been suggested (Bruch, 1974) that this is a way of changing places with a younger sib, who becomes big and plump whilst the patient becomes thin and does not grow. Certainly, acquaintances who have not seen the family for a number of months can, during the acute phase, mix them up!

The anorectic's generosity with food must be compared with her meanness with money. Starvation brings a hoarding instinct which, sadly, can be manifested in shoplifting (Crisp et al., 1980a).

The attitude of the male anorectic to his food is similar to that described above. However, male anorectics are more likely to be bulimic and more likely to abuse alcohol. The condition tends to become quickly entrenched, and the prognosis is poorer.

THE BULIMIC SYNDROME

Bingeing with food can be experienced to such an exaggerated degree that it becomes all-encompassing and life-disrupting. When at this extreme of neurotic intensity the symptom can become the central pillar around which other dietary symptoms cluster, thereby forming a syndrome—the bulimic syndrome.

This syndrome has a distinct psychopathology and occurs in patients at normal, or near normal, body weight for age and height. It is distinct from, though related to, anorexia nervosa, for such patients do not show the phobia of normal body weight which is the pathognomonic feature of anorexia nervosa (Crisp, 1967b). Neither do the patients demonstrate the essential features of anorexia nervosa as determined by Russell (1970) or Feighner et al. (1972). There is no morbid fear of becoming fat, although they do declare the normal female preoccupation with shape and weight (Nylander, 1971) as described above.

In recent years this disorder has been variously labelled. It has thus been called 'bulimorexia' (Boskind-Lodahl, 1976), 'hyperexia nervosa' (Ziolko, 1976), 'bulimia nervosa' (Russell, 1979), 'dysorexia' (Vandereycken and Pierloot, 1980), the 'bulimic syndrome' (Lacey, 1980) as well as the 'thin–fat syndrome' (Bruch, 1974), the 'dietary chaos syndrome' (Palmer, 1979) and the 'abnormal–normal weight control syndrome' (Crisp, 1981). Within the diversity of symptoms offered by such patients it would be surprising if the clinical descriptions were identical; emphasis varies, which perhaps indicates the heterogeneous nature of the condition in both its clinical presentation and its aetiology. Some authors leave it undifferentiated from bulimia occurring in an anorectic after restoration of normal body weight. To this author it seems unnecessary to change the name of the condition in such a circumstance: the patient still has anorexia nervosa, and the condition is different from bulimia occurring in a patient with no previous history of anorexia.

On presentation, the patient's initial complaint is of a turbulent pattern of eating which, by definition, includes bulimia. The inevitable weight gain which would ensue is controlled by abstinence or by laxative abuse; or by psychogenic vomiting; or by a combination of methods. If the patient is abstinent or 'dieting' then she will forbear those particular foods which will later be wolfishly over-indulged.

It is not uncommon for spouse and general practitioner to know nothing of the patient's behaviour: bulimia is a private affair. The patient usually restricts her over-eating to a 'safe' place, often a particular room in her home, where discovery of her behaviour is unlikely. The room will be locked, the telephone taken from the receiver and visitors ignored. Where the bulimia is known, attempts by friends or relatives to interrupt an attack may lead to marked anger, although sometimes friends vicariously collude or even join in!

The bulimia is periodic but chronic, with bouts becoming more frequent or more violent when the patient is emotionally stressed by interpersonal conflicts. Patterns of eating in bulimia obviously vary. Typically, however, the patient divides her days into 'good' and 'bad' days, perhaps with deeper psychological meaning. Superficially, a good day is one when she restricts her carbohydrate and calorific intake, whilst a bad day indicates a tendency to eat carbohydrates specifically, whether or not bulimia actually occurs.

Prior to the bulimic attack the patient has a feeling of expectancy, elation, or excitement associated with a compulsion to 'stuff' something into her mouth. The ingestion of the food is felt as humiliating—even in some, degrading—although the majority describe a sense of guilt which can only be expunged by vomiting. All describe being 'bloated' and over-perceive their bodies as 'gross': their descriptions implying being passive victims rather than active participants in their behaviour.

Psychogenic vomiting is not a primary symptom within this disorder: it is simply a means of preventing obesity if 'dieting' fails. Vomiting, without nausea, usually occurs after bulimia, but can follow any substantial food ingestion. It removes the 'bloated' feeling by which name the fear of aggressive obesity is often described. Vomiting is associated with a feeling of reassurance, and a determination never to binge again. Initially, it is achieved by irritating the back of the throat, or by the use of a household emetic. Later, such methods need not be employed. By standing with her head over a lavatory bowl, the patient can spontaneously induce a violent contraction of diaphragm and abdominal muscles to empty her stomach contents.

Abuse of laxatives, diuretics, or 'slimming pills' are yet other ways of preventing weight gain, or of controlling the over-perception of body shape associated with a heavy carbohydrate load. They are often used—singularly or in combination—before the patient resorts to vomiting. Perhaps for this reason they do not seem to be as emotionally laden and, consequently, are easier to give up. However, vast numbers of the tablets can be taken.

Electrolyte disturbances can occur, particularly if the patient combines the abuse of laxatives or diuretics with vomiting. The patient appears pale, sweaty, and tremulous. Usually, she will feel 'jittery', although more profound disorders can result. Fits, tetany, and pyrexia can lead to misdiagnosis. The reason for transient pyrexia, associated with bulimia, is not known but is perhaps related to the close juxtaposition of temperature and satiety 'centres' in the hypothalamus.

Menstrual irregularities are commonly associated with the bulimic syndrome. In a recent study (Lacey, 1980) of 20 patients fulfilling the criteria of the bulimic syndrome, 12 (60 per cent) described amenorrhoea of at least 10 months' duration. One subject had no menstrual bleeding, despite being on the contraceptive pill (Table 1). A further four subjects described irregular menstruation and three more described regular bleeds—these were all on the contraceptive pill. Only one subject had a normal menstrual cycle and was not on the contraceptive pill.

TABLE 1 Menstrual activity of 20 consecutive patients

	Patients affected	On 'Pill'
Amenorrhoea	12	1
Irregular menstruation	4	1
Regular 'bleeds'	3	3
Normal menstruation	1	0

Menstrual function is clearly dependent on many factors, body weight and emotional state being but two. Bulimic patients are certainly emotionally labile, but similar mental states seen in general psychiatric populations (but without an eating disorder) do not demonstrate such marked menstrual irregularity. Further, their weights, though fluctuating, are within the mean for age and height. It is noteworthy that those populations (in the Third World, etc.) whose food is high in carbohydrate, yet are in overall calorie deficit, maintain menstruation (and ovulation!) whilst bulimics who selectively avoid or manipulate carbohydrate, yet have adequate energy intake, do not. Could it be that a constant and adequate supply of carbohydrate is a necessary criterion for continuing ovulation? Whilst this hypothesis is contentious, it would make sense in evolutionary terms. The diet of primitive woman as she evolved from the Higher Apes was carbohydrate (Hawkes and Woolley, 1963).

If, therefore, carbohydrate is a major source of energy supplies to the procreatively important female fat deposits alluded to earlier, a sensitive switch, possibly hormonal, linking carbohydrate ingestion to ovulation is essential if pregnancy and lactation were not to deplete those fat stores dangerously at times of reduced food availability. Such a 'switch' would have evolutionary survival value.

In the same study, patients had moved social class during their adolescence, mainly due to education. Based on occupation, the sample tended to come from social classes I, II and III when first presenting at the clinic. This is a similar distribution to that observed in anorexia nervosa studies. However, interestingly, the social class pattern of the fathers of the patients was markedly dissimilar to that of their daughters. A total of fourteen fathers (70 per cent) came from social classes IV and V (Table 2).

TABLE 2   Social class pattern of 20 female bulimics and their fathers

Social class	Patients	Fathers of patients
1 'Professional'	1	0
2 'Intermediate'	12	1
3 'Skilled'	6	5
4 'Semi-skilled'	1	12
5 'Unskilled'	0	2
TOTALS	20	20

The social class background of the families of these patients is thus similar to the family background of massively obese populations (Silverstone, 1968). This suggests that psychogenic vomiting is a middle-class phenomenon and prevents the development of progressive and massive obesity which would otherwise have been the destiny of these patients (Lacey, in press).

Psychiatric presentation

Patients in the psychiatric clinic population tend to fall into three groups:

(1) 'Neurotic' group

This is the largest group. The patients tend to be quiet, shy women, hard-working and ambitious with high ethical standards. The predominant clinical symptom, apart from the eating disorder, is anger — although it is usually denied. Superficially, they declare sadness or depression and have often been previously diagnosed as 'reactive depressives'. A small number present with anxiety–phobic features. Such patients may describe their eating behaviour in depersonalized terms: it is as if, as an automaton, they observe their bulimic behaviour from afar, their bodies being divorced from themselves. Again, there is a barely hidden yet undeclared anger, which may be directed towards the patient herself or, more usually, a male partner or men in general.

(2) The personality disordered group

In this much smaller group manipulation of food is associated, to a varying degree, with alcohol and drug abuse. The patients 'use' them interchangeably and in a similar way. They thus binge with alcohol and describe alterations of brief bouts of grossly pathological drinking with long phases of normality, during which they are able to drink socially, or to abstain altogether. Phases of drinking, like their bulimia, may commence with explosive suddenness. A recent pilot study, with which the author is associated, intimates that 15 per cent of female alcoholics at a London clinic had a past history of eating disorders. Similar behaviour is shown towards the addictive drugs, the choice of drug depending more on their current, social acquaintances than on personal choice. In patients whose appetite behaviour is so impulsively out of control, it is not surprising that periods of sexual disinhibition occur. Many patients frankly describe this as 'promiscuity'. In others, a fear of 'going out of control' leads them to seek 'safe' relationships which can take a number of forms. Thus, the partner may be married and unprepared or unwilling to make a commitment, or he may be held in such low esteem by the patient that the relationship has little intrinsic worth. Sometimes the partner may be homosexual or bisexual, or simply described by the patient as 'weak'. Fellatio may be the sole and exclusive form of sexual intercourse. Temporary and brief prostitution is resorted to by a small number. Occasionally, the partner may be female, and homosexuality tends to be used as a protection — a way of seeking sexual release without meaningful commitment or future. Clinically, such patients may present as emotionally shallow or histrionic. Superficial wrist-cutting or burning the skin with cigarette stubs can occur. The more verbal patients will describe this as a mortification of the flesh. The clinical presentation of this group is thus markedly dissimilar from the vast majority of bulimic patients, described above.

(3) The epileptiform group

In a small number of patients the bulimic syndrome occurs in, and is generated by, diagnosable epilepsy. It should be emphasized that the fits are not secondary to the vomiting and laxative abuse, occurring as a result of electrolyte imbalance, but are primary. Such patients describe epileptiform fits or 'absences' which pre-date the eating disorder. A constant feature in the history of these patients is that the first epileptic fit took place within the context of puberty: the normal insecurities of that time being heightened by the lack of control intrinsic within a fit. Diagnosis needs to be based on a clear history of fits pre-dating the bulimia or psychogenic vomiting, or the presence of epileptiform phenomena following resolution of the abnormal dietary behaviour.

Aetiology and pathogenesis

Although the aetiology and attitude towards food of the two main groups of bulimics are similar, some differences do occur.

Abnormal eating behaviour in the neurotic group usually starts within the context of the failure of the patient's first major sexual relationship, or following a series of brief, but abortive, relationships. The patient, wounded, examines herself critically and feels very low in self-esteem. She feels a failure as a woman and projects this failure on to her body shape. By dieting and altering her shape she feels she can alter herself but quickly stumbles into bulimia, a symptom which reinforces her sense of failure. Sometimes the bulimia begins during pregnancy, or in the puerperium: usually such patients doubt their maternal feelings and find themselves struggling and depressed while caring for their new infant. Again, the pattern of eating behaviour is associated with the feeling of being a failure; in all cases the patient seems to be struggling to achieve a perfect, yet stereotyped, feminine role.

The seeds of the bulimic eating derive from the emotional turmoil of late adolescence and the movement of social class by education which are persistent features. Attempting to identify with the slimmer body shape and lower body weight of their middle-class schoolgirl peers, they begin to relate social and emotional security with carbohydrate abstention. 'Dieting', or more accurately carbohydrate avoidance, is seen as a means of bringing control to the chaos they feel in and around their lives. They link their body shape (and weight) emotionally and socially to their sexuality, a matter about which these patients are so unsure; and their body shape and its manipulation become all-preoccupying. Logically, as they see it, the manipulation of shape and weight becomes the answer to any major emotional stress. The syndrome seems to be a clear extension of the compulsive eating which is common in late adolescent middle-class girls and as a means of thwarting obesity which would, perhaps, have been their destiny if they had remained within their parents' social class.

The personality-disordered group feel that their eating pattern is out of control. This lack of control may extend to the abuse of alcohol or other drugs and, also, to other appetites, particularly their sexual drives. The patient finds the lack of meaning for long-term commitment within her relationship reassuring, safe, and uncomplicated; her own doubts being dealt with by humiliation of her more passive partner. The humiliation or devaluation of the sexual partner (or herself) seems to be a part of a desperate attempt to deny feelings of dependence. So interrelated is bulimia and sexual activity in the minds of such patients that they may use intercourse or masturbation as a means of thwarting a bulimic attack or, alternatively, gorging to sedation may be used to lower heightened sexual drive.

All the patients, of whatever group, are fascinated and haunted by food, particularly carbohydrate. Some use it, in excess, as a sedative to calm the sense of loss they feel in and around their lives, such that it develops an addictive quality. Others use it to cheapen and degrade themselves: an affront associated with guilt and secrecy. All declare marked unsureness of their femininity, together with overwhelming difficulties in their interpersonal relationships. These feelings are related, both temporally and psychodynamically, by the patient herself to the eating symptoms which first led her to seek help.

OBESITY

Few animals have been given such free access to 'nutritious' food, so appetizingly presented, as modern Western man; and few animals have enjoyed such indolence! If man has inherited mechanisms and controls developed from a more austere world it would, indeed, be astounding if he were not prone to obesity (Tudge, 1977).

Obesity thus presents yet another response to food. The overwhelming majority of obese people become fat because of an individual and variable mixture of psychological and sociocultural factors, with possible genetic and metabolic influences as well. Obesity is a state of excessive fatness which is usually defined by clinicians in terms of some degree of 'being over-weight'. There is no absolute measure of obesity: it is necessary to construe the term 'excessive fatness' within the context of the population being examined.

In *infancy*, obesity may be a reflection of the eating habits of the mother as well as the constitution of both parents. The relationship between the obese child and his mother seems to be quantitatively different from that of a normal-weight child. A mother with both normal and obese children appears to feed them differently, and even when advised by a physician to the contrary, may persist in giving excessive helpings to her over-weight offspring (Bruch, 1943; Dunbar, 1954; Crisp, 1967). Food tends to be an emotional item between mother and child, and the relationship between them can be ambiguous and ambivalent.

There continues to be marked disagreement between investigators about the importance of emotional factors in childhood obesity—whether they contribute to its development or whether the psychological problems are secondary to the social rejection obese youngsters encounter (Bruch, 1974). Most probably the two aspects are intertwined.

Kalucy (1976) has summarized four features peculiar to the families of obese youngsters. First, food can be a primary or major means of giving and receiving affection, or of relieving distress, or of rewarding desired behaviour. Holding and cuddling are less used than the giving of food. Second, the mother tends to respond to discomfort with food, and this, Kalucy suggests, would tend to diminish the child's capacity to distinguish hunger from more appropriate responses. The child tends not to develop the responses to stress, to fear, or to excitement that a normal-weight child would learn. Third, the family's attitude to meals and food is rigid. Thus, the child receives instruction that all served food must be eaten. Such rigidity can lead to a diminished ability to recognize hunger and to initiate and cease eating according to need (Bychowski, 1950). Fourth, many of the mother's feelings and responses to the child are determined by her own anxiety, uncertainty, or narcissistic needs. The effects of this is to 'confuse the subtle reinforcing experiences concerned with the relationship between hunger, fulness and one's own developing autonomy'.

Work deriving from the National Survey of Child Development (Crisp *et al.*, 1970) suggests that 'fat' infants tend to remain plump as children and adolescents. The National Survey involved a prospective nationwide study of a cohort of 5362 babies born during the first week of March 1946 and investigated at that time and also subsequently—mainly at the ages of 4, 7, 11, and 15. Of the 240 boys who were fat at 7 years of age, only seven were thin at 15 years, and of the 243 girls who were fat at 7, only three had become thin at 15. The Survey also suggested that fatter children tend to be the first born or the youngest sibling within a family. Somewhat surprisingly, perhaps, fat children tended to give a history of being breast-fed and social class was not found to be related to adolescent obesity. The mothers of fat children expressed strikingly less anxiety about their children's health, appetite, and size than did the mothers of thin children. There was also an association between fatness in boys and aggressiveness (thinness being associated with nervousness).

Thus, when examined over a decade or so, most people show remarkable stability of body weight. Minor fluctuation is, of course, usual, as is the tendency to gain some weight with the passing years. Yet, the energy imbalance which generates these changes is minuscule when put within the context of the vast amount of energy which is consumed and expended during this time. Most people, therefore, have within themselves a control mechanism which, whilst not exquisitely fine, is at least adequate.

What then, are the characteristics of those who cannot maintain their weight? It is necessary to remind ourselves that there appear to be major differences between the obese in the general community and the minority who declare themselves patients and seek help in our clinics. Their characteristics are different, and it would be wrong to project the problems, symptoms, and prognosis of the clinic patients on to a non-clinic population, even if the two groups were of similar weight.

Few general population studies have been done. In the downtown Manhattan study little association was found between psychiatric status and obesity (Moore et al., 1962). However Simon (1963) found significantly less depression amongst obese Service personnel than amongst non-obese colleagues. Similarly, Silverstone (1968) reported that men who were 45 per cent above 'ideal' body weight and sampled from a general population were less neurotic than a normal-weight control group. Moreover, Crisp and McGuinness (1976) found massive obesity in a general practice population in south-west London to be associated with significantly less anxiety and depression. In general, there is evidence that people who are moderately over-weight—say up to 50 per cent above ideal weight—are less emotionally disturbed than those who are nearer the mean weight for their age and height, and certainly so when compared with those who are thin.

However, that sub-group of people who present themselves to the obesity clinics are very different. The clinic population, which tends to be self-selected, is marked by being female and having a severe, usually progressive, decompensating obesity and by being markedly neurotic (Crisp, 1978).

Prolonged dietary restriction with weight loss in the obese leads to change in mood, particularly depression (Bruch, 1957; Stunkard, 1957) or a variety of psychotic reactions (Robinson and Winnik, 1973). In contrast, Kalucy and Crisp (1974) and Solow et al. (1974) found that patients who achieved substantial weight loss by surgery showed little tendency to develop depression. Two factors may be relevant in interpreting this finding. First, patients who have had bypass surgery are not food-deprived in the same way as those who severely restrict their diet. Second, surgery is unlikely to lead to a weight loss of more than one-third of the initial presenting weight and so the patient remains moderately obese (Pilkington, 1981). This residual obesity may be important psychologically for it has been claimed that obesity acts as a barrier—a protection which allows the patient to deny interpersonal problems (Crisp, 1978). Certainly, major weight loss leads to much emotional disturbance, as these repressed difficulties can no longer be avoided. Crisp suggests there is a critical weight threshold (being about 25 per cent above normal weight) below which such denial is no longer achieved. The threshold also marks the limit of sexual quiescence which is a feature of massive obesity, as it is of abstaining anorexia nervosa. This threshold is certainly more diffuse than those found at a lower body weight (see above) but there is evidence that it, too, is hormonally determined (Kalucy, 1976).

Certainly, massive obesity is important in the promotion and maintenance of sexual inactivity: it may be used in the resolution of sexual conflict and treatment may, therefore, have major implications to the marital relationship. It should also be recalled that most massively obese women marry when they are grossly over-weight, and therefore the marriage was decided within the context of that obesity and its implications.

The author has also noted, during psychotherapy, how some female massively obese patients, whose obesity occurred apparently without reason, can describe how they suddenly found themselves the object of incestuous attention at about the time of puberty, and how rapid progressive obesity led not only to a reduction of sexual molestation but also to a reduction in their own emerging sexual impulsivity. They feared that this impulsivity was responsible for the 'unwanted' attention.

The eating patterns of obese patients are highly variable. Most over-eat at times of emotional stress, but otherwise eat fewer calories and have fewer meals each day than do people of normal weight (Rose and Williams, 1961; Fabry, 1969; Schachter, 1971; Hawkins, 1979). However, bulimic eating does occur, but it is characteristic of only a minority. Thus, Stunkard (1959) found it in only 8 per cent of his clinic study. Hamburger (1951), however, reported it in all of his small sample—but these were psychotherapy cases and highly selected.

Self-induced vomiting is rarely mentioned in the literature but does occur— the author has a number of obese patients who intermittently vomit under emotional stress, but this vomiting is not enough to reduce their body weight to the normal range (and hence enter the 'bulimic syndrome').

It was Schachter (1971) who stated that the trigger of the eating response in the obese was different from people of normal body weight: the obese respond to more 'external' pressures such as the availability of food than to 'internal' experiences such as hunger. However, Nisbett (1972) modified this by noting that anyone attempting to enforce their weight below their personal physio- logical 'set-point' weight was susceptible to the undue influence of external factors such as the sight, taste, and smell of food or the sight of others eating, and that this was not restricted to the obese alone. Nisbett proposed that the 'set-point' threshold was maintained by the hypothalamus and that people who attempted to diet below it will always be 'physiologically hungry'. In other words, because the 'set-point' or threshold level of fat tissue is variable in the population, certain people have a biological destiny to be fat. However, it would be trite to claim that cognition does not play a major role in the short- term regulation of food intake. Polivy (1976) demonstrated that subjects who were dieting were more likely to over-eat after a 'pre-load' which they believed was high in calories, or following emotional distress, or alcohol.

FOOD AND OTHER MOOD STATES

The infant's preoccupation with its mouth suggested to the early analysts that orality was the first 'stage' of emotional gratification in the process of personality development. Difficulties at any 'stage' could lead to arrested development. Thus the psychoanalytic movement ascribed neurotic eating difficulties to trauma at an early stage of development. Pathological 'eating' problems are judged to be the residual symptom in a personality predominantly fused or arrested in the oral stage (Alexander, 1934; Bruch, 1952; Stunkard, 1958; Rubin, 1968). Such a theory, based on anecdotal clinical findings, has its critics (Glucksman and Hirsch, 1968), but it is nonetheless common and is derived from intense and skilled clinical enquiry.

The oral stage, an analytical terms the earliest, is the essence of the mother–child relationship, and it suggested to analysts that mother love—both in its presence and absence—becomes equated symbolically with eating.

During the first few months of life the developing infant, given normal maternal security, pursues a sleep–wakefulness cycle governed mainly by his nutritional needs. Some infants adjust quickly to sleeping through the night, whilst others put up much resistance. The view is held that the depressive state stems from unresolved conflict around this time, caused by the partial withdrawal of the mother and her food supply. A sense of loss and rejection, and even a state of depression, thus becomes associated with hunger and wakefulness (Alexander, 1934; Hamburger, 1951; Bruch, 1952; Glucksman and Hirsch, 1968).

Food manipulation and weight fluctuation occur in association with any psychiatric illness. However, compensatory eating is very common in mild, neurotic depression, whilst a reduced appetite is frequent in the more endogenous (biological) depressions. If reduced appetite leads to substantial weight loss then the 'characteristic' early-morning wakening occurs. This sleep disturbance is not intrinsic to the disorder, but seems to be a function of the weight loss itself (see anorexia nervosa). Schizophrenics rarely manipulate food, although weight gain is a frequent side-effect of phenothiazine medication (Paykel et al., 1978). Weight loss also occurs in hypomania. The patient declares a poor appetite but this needs to be judged within the characteristic manic excitement, fleeting attention span, and hyperactivity.

CONCLUSION

Attitudes to food are rarely simple. Although biological at root, the processes of evolutional and social change have led to food being associated with bizarre behaviours and beliefs. Various psychological and psychopathological patterns have developed which are the subject of intense recent and ongoing research.

REFERENCES

Alexander, F. (1934). The influence of psychological factors upon gastrointestinal disturbances. *Psychoanal. Q.*, 3, 501–12.

Armstrong-Esther, C. A., Lacey, J. H., Crisp, A. H., and Bryant, T. N. (1978). An investigation of the immune response of patients suffering from anorexia nervosa. *Postgrad. Med. J.*, **54**, 395-9.

Berry Brazelton, T. (1976). *Toddlers and Parents*. Macmillan, London.

Boskind-Lodahl, M. (1976). Cinderella's stepsisters: a feminist perspective on anorexia nervosa and bulimia. *Signs*, **2**, 342-56.

Brook, C. G. D. (1981). Endocrinological control of growth at puberty. In: *Control of Growth* (ed. J. M. Tanner). Churchill Livingstone, London.

Bruch, H. (1943). Psychiatric aspects of obesity in children. *Am. J. Psychiatry*, **99**, 752.

Bruch, H. (1952). Psychologic aspects of reducing. *Psychosom. Med.* 14, 337-41.

Bruch, H. (1957). *The Importance of Overweight*. Norton, New York.

Bruch, H. (1965). The psychiatric differential diagnosis of anorexia nervosa. In: *Symposium on Anorexia Nervosa*, Gottinger, Thième, Verlag, Stuttgart.

Bruch, H. (1974). *Eating Disorders*. Routledge & Kegan Paul, London.

Bychowski, G. (1950). A neurotic obesity. *Psychoanal. Rev.*, **37**, 301-8.

Cleghorn, R. A., and Brown, W. T. (1964). Eating patterns and nutritional adaptation. *Can. Psychiat. Assoc. J.*, **9**, 299.

Crisp, A. H. (1967a). "Anorexia nervosa". *Hosp. Med*, **1**, 713-18.

Crisp, A. H. (1967b). The possible significance of some behavioural correlates of weight and carbohydrate intake. *J. Psychosom. Res.*, **11**, 117-26.

Crisp, A. H. (1977). The differential diagnosis of anorexia nervosa. *Proc. R. Soc. Med.*, **70**, 231-8.

Crisp, A. H. (1978). Some psychosomatic aspects of obesity. In: *Recent Advances in Obesity Research*, vol. II (ed. G. Bray). Newman, London.

Crisp, A. H. (1981). Anorexia nervosa at normal body weight! The abnormal normal weight control syndrome. *Int. J. Psychiat. Med.*, **11** (3), 203-33.

Crisp, A. H. and McGuiness, B. (1976). Jolly fat: the relationship between obesity and psychoneurosis in the general population. *Br. Med. J.*, **1**, 7-9.

Crisp, A. H. and Kalucy, R. S. (1974). Aspects of the perceptual disorder in anorexia nervosa. *Br. J. Med. Psychol.*, **47**, 349-61.

Crisp, A. H., Douglas, J. W. B., Ross, J. M., and Stone-Hill, E. (1970). Some developmental aspects of disorders of weight. *J. Psychosom. Res.*, **14**, 313.

Crisp, A. H., Hsu, L. K. G., and Harding, B. (1980a). The starving hoarder and voracious spender. Stealing in anorexia nervosa. *J. Psychosom. Res.*, **24**, 225-31.

Crisp, A. H., Hsu, L. K. G. and Harding, B. (1980b). The long term prognosis in anorexia nervosa: some factors predictive of outcome. In: *Anorexia Nervosa* (ed. R. A. Vigersky). Raven Press, New York.

Dally, P. (1969). *Anorexia Nervosa*. Wm. Heinemann, London.

DHSS (1975). A nutrition survey of pre-school children, 1967-68. *Report on Health and Social Subjects*, 10.

Dunbar, F. (1954). *Emotions and Bodily Changes*. Columbia University Press, New York.

Fabry, P. (1969). *Eating Patterns and Nutritional Adaptation*. Butterworths, London.

Feighner, J. P., Robins, E., Guze, S. B., Woodruff, R. A., Winclur, G., and Munoz, R. (1972). Diagnostic criteria for use in psychiatric research. *Arch. Gen. Psychiatry*, **26**, 57-63.

Frisch, R. E. and McArthur, J. W. (1974). Menstrual cycles, fatness as a determinant of minimum weight for height necessary for their maintenance or onset. *Science*, **185**, 949-51.

Garner, D. M., Garfinkel, P. E., Schwartz, D ., and Thompson, M. (1980). Cultural expectations of thinness in women, *Psychol. Rep.*, **47**, 483-91.

Glucksman, M. L., and Hirsch, J. (1968). The response of obese patients to weight reduction: a clinical evaluation of behaviour. *Psychosom. Med.*, **30**, 1–8.

Hamburger, W. W . (1951). Emotional aspects of obesity. *Med. Clin. N. Am.*, **35**, 483–99.

Hawkes, J. and Woolley, Sir L. (1963). *Prehistory and the Beginnings of Civilisation*. George Allen & Unwin, London.

Hawkins, R. C. (1979). Meal/snack frequencies of College Students: a normative study. *Behav. Psychother.*, **7**, 85–9.

Huenemann, R. L., and Turner, O. (1942). Methods of dietary investigation. *J. Am. Diet. Assoc.*, **18**, 562–8.

Huenemann, R. L., Shapiro, L. R., Hampton, M. C., and Mitchell, B. W. (1966). A longitudinal study of gross body composition and body conformation and their association with food and activity in a teenage population. *Am. J. Clin. Nutr.*, **18**, 325–38.

Hurst, P. S., Lacey, J. H., and Crisp, A. H. (1977). Teeth, vomiting and diet: a study of the dental characteristics of seventeen anorexia nervosa patients. *Postgrad. Med. J.*, **53**, 298–305.

Kalucy, R. S. (1976). Obesity: an attempt to find a common ground among some of the biological, psychological and sociological phenomenon of obesity/overeating syndromes. In: *Psychosomatic Approach to the prevention of disease* (Proceedings) (ed. M. Carruthers and. R. Priest). Pergamon Press, Oxford.

Kalucy, R. S., and Crisp, A. H. (1974). Some psychological and social implications of massive obesity. *J. Psychosom. Res.*, **18**, 465–73.

Lacey, J. H. (1980). 'The bulimic syndrome'. *Proceedings 13th European Congress of Psychosomatic Research, Istanbul.*

Lacey, J. H. (in press). 'The bulimic syndrome at normal body weight: reflections on pathogenesis and clinical features'. *Int. J. Eating Disorders.*

Lacey, J. H., Chadbund, C., Crisp, A. H., Whithead, J., and Stordy, J. (1978). Variation in energy intake of adolescent girls. *J. Human Nutr.*, **32**, 419–26.

Lacey, J. H., Crisp, A. H., Hart, G., and Kirkwood, B. A. (1979). Weight and skeletal maturation—a study of radiological and chronological age in an anorexia nervosa population. *Postgrad. Med. J.*, **55**, 381–5.

Lacey, J. H., Crisp, A. H., Kalucy, R. S., Hartmann, M. K., and Chen, C. N. (1975). Weight gain and the sleeping electroencephalogram: study of 10 patients with anorexia nervosa. *Br. Med. J.*, 6 December, pp.556–8.

Moore, M. A., Stundard, A. J., and Srole, L. (1962). Obesity, social class and mental illness. *J. Am. Med. Assoc.*, **181**, 962.

Nemiah, J. C. (1958). Anorexia nervosa: fact and theory. *Am. J. Dig. Dis.*, **3**, 249–251.

Nisbett, R. E. (1972). Hunger, obesity and the ventromedial hypothalamus. *Psychol. Rev.*, **79**, 434–453.

Nylander, I. (1971). The feeling of being fat and dieting in a school population: an epidemiologic interview investigation. *Acta Socio-Medica Scand.*, **3**, 17–26.

Orbach, S. (1978). *Fat is a Feminist Issue*. Paddington Press, London.

Palmer, R. L. (1979). The dietary chaos syndrome; a useful new term?. *Br. J. Med. Psychol.*, **52**, 187–90.

Palmer, R. L., Crisp, A. H., Mackinnon, P. C. B., Franklin, M., Bonnar, J., and Wheeler, M. (1975). Pituitary sensitivity to 50 µg LH/FSH-RH in subjects with anorexia nervosa in acute and recovery stages. *Br. Med. J.*, **1**, 179–82.

Paykel, E. S. (1977). Depression and appetite. *J. Psychosom. Res.*, **21**, 401–7.

Pilkington, T. R. E. (1980). Weight loss following intestinal bypass. In: *Surgical*

Management of Obesity (eds J. D. Maxwell, J.-C. Gazet, and T. R. E. Pilkington). Academic Press, London.

Polivy, J. (1976). Perception of calories and regulation of intake in restrained and unrestrained subjects. *Addict. Behav.*, 1, 237–43.

Robinson, S. and Winnick, H. (1973). Severe psychotic disturbance following crash diet weight loss. *Arch. Gen. Psychiatry*, 29, 559–64.

Rose, G. A., and Williams, T. R. (1961). Metabolic studies on large and small eaters. *Br. J. Nutr.*, 15, 1–9.

Rubin, R. (1968). Body image and self-esteem. *Nursing Outlook*, 16, 20–4.

Russell, G. F. M. (1970). Anorexia nervosa—its identity as an illness and its treatment. In: *Modern Trends in Psychological Medicine* (ed. J. H. Price), vol. 2, pp.131–64. Butterworth, London.

Russell, G. F. M. (1979). Bulimia nervosa: an ominous variant of anorexia nervosa. *Psychol. Med.*, 9, 429–48.

Russell, G. F. M., and Beardwood, C. J. (1968). The feeding disorders with particular reference to anorexia nervosa and its associated gonadotrophic changes. In: *Endocrinology and Human Behaviour* (ed. R. P. Michael). Oxford University Press, London.

Schachter, S. (1971). *Emotion, Obesity and Crime*. Academic Press, New York.

Silverstone, J. T. (1968). Psychological aspects of obesity. *Proc. R. Soc. Med.*, 61, 371–8.

Simon, R. I. (1963). Obesity as a depressive equivalent. *J. Am. Med. Assoc.*, 182, 108.

Solow, C., Silverfarb, P. M., and Swift, K. (1974). Effects of intestinal bypass surgery for obesity. *N. Engl. J. Med.*, 290, 300–5.

Stunkard, A. J. (1957). The dieting depression. *Am. J. Med.*, 23, 77–82.

Stunkard, A. J. (1958). Physical activity, emotions and human obesity. *Psychosom. Med.*, 20, 366.

Stunkard, A. J. (1959). Eating patterns and obesity. *Psychiat. Q.*, 33, 284–92.

Thoma, H. (1967). *Anorexia Nervosa* (trans. Gilliam Brydone) International University Press, New York.

Thomson, A. M. (1958). Diet in pregnancy. *Br. J. Nutr.*, 12, 446–61.

Tudge, C. (1977). Fat and ignorance. *World Med.*, 10, 29–38.

Vandereycken, W., and Pierloot, R. (1980). Dysorexia: bulimia and anorexia nervosa. *Proceedings 13th European Conference on Psychosomatic Research, Istanbul*.

Widdowson, E. M., and McCance, R. A. (1936). A study of English diets by the individual method. II: women. *J. Hyg.*, 36, 293–309.

Yudkin, J. (1951). Dietary surveys: variation in the weekly intake of nutrients. *Br. J. Nutr.*, 4, 177–94.

Ziolko, H. U. (1976). Hyperexia nervosa. *Psychother. Med. Psycha*, 26, 10–12.

Clinical Reactions to Food
Edited by M. H. Lessof
© 1983 John Wiley & Sons Ltd.

Immunology and Physiology of Digestion

Anne Ferguson

Reader in Medicine (Gastroenterology)
University of Edinburgh

and

Stephan Strobel

Research Fellow
University of Frankfurt

INTRODUCTION

The digestive tract of man has a remarkable capacity to adapt to different patterns of eating as well as to the enormous variety of foods which are consumed. There are complex mechanisms for the regulation of digestion, and the autonomic nervous system, circulating hormones, and local neural and endocrine tissues in the wall of the gut integrate to control gut motility, secretion of digestive juices, absorption of nutrients, and elimination of residue. Regulatory mechanisms also exist for the induction and suppression of immunological reactions to the antigens of ingested foods.

It is impossible to separate the digestive and immunological functions of the gut (Figure 1). Whereas most of the cells of the body are in a sterile environment and are exposed to only a limited number of antigens, the gastrointestinal epithelium separates the tissues of the body from a very large number of living and non-living antigens, the majority of which are harmless and indeed may even be beneficial to the host. The nature and amounts of digestive secretions, speed of onward propulsion or intestinal stasis, rapidity of absorption and of elimination will all influence — by dilution, neutralization, or excretion — the amounts of antigen present in a particular segment of the gut. For example in pancreatic insufficiency, when protein digestion is impaired, there will be much greater quantities than normal of immunogenic

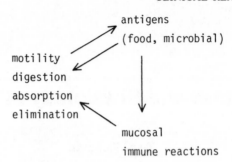

FIGURE 1   Complex interrelationships between the digestive functions of the gut, intestinal antigens and immune responses.

dietary material presented to the jejunum and ileum. When an intestinal mucosal disease results from immune reactions to antigens such as foods or micro-organisms, the length of the gut affected by disease will be directly related to the distribution of the antigen within the intestine. On the other hand disturbances in secretions and in motility will influence the microbial flora of the proximal small intestine. In achlorhydria, which frequently accompanies hypogammaglobulinaemia, the minimum infectious dose of bacteria is reduced and the patient is at risk of developing bacterial colonization of the proximal intestine.

It has been necessary for the mucosal immune system to develop a remarkable flexibility. Against the background of continuous low-grade specific immune responses to food antigens and commensal bacteria, the gut allows the passage of nutritious substances and tolerates the presence of many useful micro-organisms, but retains the capacity to mount a range of protective immune responses to enteric pathogens, which have the effect of eliminating infection and preventing re-infection.

Mucosal immunological reactions contribute to tissue immunity and also to the neutralization and degradation of antigens. These immune reactions also profoundly influence gastrointestinal structure and function, as discussed below. A further dimension to the complexity of this series of interrelating facets of the gut is the fact that some of the effects of immune responses to bacteria and parasites are very similar to the effects which may be produced directly by parasite or microbial toxins—for example alterations in epithelial cell kinetics with villous atrophy and crypt hyperplasia, secretion of mucus, and increased permeability to macromolecules.

Surprisingly, many digestive functions remain normal even in patients with severe gastrointestinal disease, and so do the majority of immunological responses to foodstuffs. It is only exceptionally that a patient with oesophageal, gastric, pancreatic, intestinal or liver disease cannot tolerate a full diet. When this is so, often only a simple modification of the diet will be required to relieve food-related symptoms—a low-residue diet for patients with stricturing lesions of the intestines, or a low-fat diet in patients with steatorrhoea. Against this background it is surprising that many individuals who have no evidence of gastrointestinal or immunological pathology complain that foodstuffs which they ingest lead to adverse clinical reactions — by definition, food intolerance. Nevertheless, subtle alterations in the digestive or immunological functions of the gut may underlie such symptoms in a proportion of patients. Depending on the mechanism, treatment may be dietary, pharmacological (related to digestive or immunological functions) or, often, no treatment may be necessary.

For that small minority of patients and diseases in whom food intolerance has been fully documented, and in whom the mechanism has been established to be immunological, the primary pathophysiological event must be seen as being a breakdown in the normal homeostatic processes of intestinal immunity. Normally, immune responses to ingested foodstuffs are harmless. Recently it has become clear that immune responses at mucosal surfaces are largely conditioned by immunoregulatory T cells. This renders it at least theoretically possible that the normal immune response could be re-established in such food-allergic individuals, by using tailored immunotherapy to manipulate the immunoregulatory cells themselves.

In this chapter we outline some aspects of the immunology and physiology of the gastrointestinal tract, with the aim of providing a background for the subsequent discussions of clinical food intolerance. Detailed descriptions of the physiology of digestion can be obtained from any textbook of physiology or gastroenterology, and so the greatest emphasis has been on the functions of the gastrointestinal immune system, and on interrelationships between digestive function and immune responses.

GASTROINTESTINAL IMMUNE APPARATUS

Gut-associated lymphoid tissues (GALT)

Investigation of the clinical immunology of the gastrointestinal tract has developed more slowly than that of systemic immunology—mainly because gastrointestinal secretions and tissues are relatively inaccessible. However it is now clear that the gut-associated lymphoid tissues (GALT) and other mucosa-associated lymphoid tissues (MALT) such as those of the lungs and the genital tract react to provoking substances (antigen) in a manner completely different and quite separate from the reaction of systemic immune systems to the same antigen. The GALT comprises nodular lymphoid tissues within the wall of the gut (e.g. Peyer's patches) and in the mesentery (mesenteric lymph nodes); the phagocytic system of the liver; many single lymphoid cells scattered throughout the mucosae and possibly even within the lumen; immunoglobulins, locally secreted and derived from the serum; and many non-specific humoral and cellular effector mechanisms such as lysozyme, mucus, and macrophages. The continuous traffic of lymphocytes, with homing of immunoblasts from the nodular lymphoid tissues of the gut via lymph and blood back to the mucosa of small bowel and colon, allows for widespread distribution of antibody-producing cells and T blasts reacting with enteric antigens. Thus the capacity for specific immune reactions to antigen is spread throughout the length of the gut, a logical phenomenon in view of the motility and reproductive capacity of many enteric pathogens.

Nodular lymphoid tissues

Peyer's patches are readily visible to the naked eye as nodules interrupting the smooth mucosal surface of the intestines. In histological sections Peyer's patches appear to comprise a number of nodules of large lymphocytes connected by sheets of small lymphocytes, with an overlying epithelium. However studies of lymphocyte types within this tissue have shown that just as in the case of lymph nodes and spleen, there are segregated T and B cell areas within the Peyer's patches, with the internodular zones and the subepithelial areas being rich in T cells (Parrott and Ferguson, 1974; Parrott, 1976). The lymphoid nodules are covered by a specialized columnar epithelium which contains few or no Paneth cells or goblet cells, but within which there are many specialized M or microfold cells, as well as enterocytes (Figure 2) (Owen

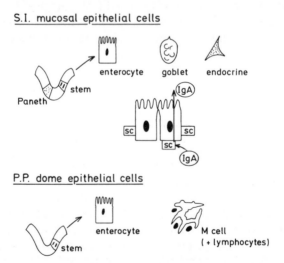

FIGURE 2   Cell types within the mucosa of the small intestine. On the villi, enterocytes, goblet cells, Paneth cells and possibly endocrine cells are produced by mitosis in the crypts of Lieberkühn. The enterocytes of the Peyer's patch dome epithelium are also derived from stem cells in adjoining crypts. The source of M cells is unknown.
PP — Peyer's patch; SC — secretory component; SI — small intestine.

and Jones, 1974). Within this relatively 'bare' part of the epithelium, M cells are ideally placed for their proposed function of antigen absorption and presentation to lymphocytes (Owen, 1977).

Single lymphoid cells in the mucosae

Many individual lymphoid cells are dispersed within the mucosae of the entire gastrointestinal tract, both within the lamina propria and intraepithelially. The maximum density of these cells is in the small intestine with relatively fewer in the colonic and gastric mucosae. Cell types include small, medium and large lymphocytes, plasma cells of all five immunoglobulin classes, mononuclear phagocytes, eosinophils, mast cells, and the occasional polymorphonuclear leucocyte. The majority of intraepithelial cells are lymphocytes but all the cell types mentioned above may be present in the lamina propria.

IE lymphocytes

There has been considerable interest recently in the nature of mucosal lymphocytes (Ferguson, 1977a). A proportion of intraepithelial (IE) lymphocytes in animals contain small granules which resemble those of mast cells although they are smaller (Guy-Grand et al., 1978). By using techniques such as immunofluorescence and peroxidase labelling with anti-T cell sera, the majority of IE lymphocytes have been shown to be T cells (Selby et al., 1981b). In a recent study of T cell subclass distribution within the gut, the majority of IE lymphocytes in man were found to be 'OKT8 positive'—that is, they stain with antisera which also stain the peripheral blood cytotoxic/suppressor T cell subclass (Selby et al., 1981a; see also Figure 7). However there is some preliminary evidence from studies in rats and mice that the IE lymphocytes are a heterogeneous population and that granulated IE lymphocytes may be unique in their cell surface marker properties.

Lamina propria plasma cells

Plasma cells are densely packed around the crypts with relatively fewer being found within the villus lamina propria. The approximate proportions of plasma cells containing immunoglobins A, M, and G (IgA, IgM, and IgG) in normal human small bowel are 82, 16, and 2 per cent and their numbers and proportions vary considerably in inflammatory diseases of the intestines (Brandtzaeg and Baklien, 1976).

Mast cells

Mucosal mast cells can be detected in the normal small intestine if appropriate fixative and staining techniques are used (Strobel et al., 1981); these mast cells differ in their staining properties and also probably in their functions, when compared with connective tissue mast cells. An occasional intraepithelial mast cell or eosinophil is observed, even in normal tissues.

Immunoglobulin E (IgE) cells

Intestinal mucosal cells which are stained by anti-IgE antisera are a subject of some dispute. Some of the earlier studies probably utilized antisera which were not completely specific for IgE and therefore have to be discounted. There seems little doubt that some of the IgE-staining cells are indeed plasma cells, although there is evidence from the rat that mucosal mast cells contain IgE (Mayrhofer, 1977). Despite these reservations, recent work by Rosekrans and his colleagues is convincing, and suggests that in some patients with gastrointestinal or food-allergic reactions, there are increased numbers of mucosal IgE-containing cells (Rosekrans *et al.*, 1980a,b). Since the mucosal IgE cell counts in normal individuals appear to be extremely low, the detection of these cells has potential as a method for diagnosis of an intestinal allergic state, and this interesting work from Holland awaits confirmation.

Traffic of intestinal lymphocytes

Small T and B lymphocytes leave the bloodstream in the post-capillary venules of Peyer's patches, to 'home' to the T and B areas of these tissues in the same pattern as they home in other organized lymphoid tissues (Parrott, 1976). The traffic route of the large T and B lymphocytes (immunoblasts) of the lymph draining Peyer's patches and mesenteric lymph nodes is quite different. There is considerable evidence from animal work that these cells home back to the gastrointestinal tract mucosa (e.g. Husband and Gowans, 1978; Guy-Grand *et al.*, 1978). This gut-seeking property of immunoblasts is not antigen-specific, for these cells will traffic to pieces of intestine from newborn animals, and to transplanted grafts of intestine which have never contained bacterial or food antigens. They also home to other MALT mucosae, such as the bronchial mucosa and the mammary gland.

Immunoglobulin A (IgA)

Intestinal secretions are rich in IgA, but also contain small amounts of IgM and IgG. These immunoglobulins are in the main derived from plasma cells within the mucosae, although there is likely to be some contribution by leakage from the serum. The structure of the secretory IgA molecule is now established and is as illustrated in Figure 3. The molecule may be found in different tissues and secretions as a 7S monomer, 10S dimer, or 11S dimer associated with secretory component. The functions played by IgA in the gut lumen are still

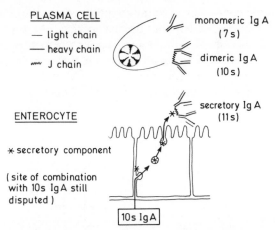

FIGURE 3   Components of a secretory IgA molecules. Monomeric IgA comprises two light and two heavy chains; in dimeric IgA, two 7S units are joined by a J chain, also synthesized in the plasma cell. Secretory component is added to 10S IgA as it passes through epithelial cells.

uncertain (Bazin, 1976). This immunoglobulin acts as an efficient agglutinating antibody and may restrict bacterial growth by blocking bacterial adherent to mucus surfaces. IgA antibodies can also combine with and neutralize toxins, and may inactivate viruses. However the presence of IgA is not essential for health, for many IgA-deficient individuals are entirely normal and have no apparent susceptibility to infectious or other diseases. The minority of IgA-deficient persons who have associated infection have recently been found to be deficient in a subclass of immunoglobulin G, IgG2 (Oxelius et al., 1981).

Of relevance to the subject of this book are the postulated functions of IgA as blocking antibodies in intestinal hypersensitivity reactions, and as agents to reduce uptake of large molecules across the intestinal mucosa (Walker and Isselbacher, 1977; Stokes et al., 1975).

IgA and the liver

An interesting series of observations has recently been made in the rat and in several other species (Figure 4). Dimeric IgA 10S, without secretory component, has been found to be selectively transported across the hepatic parenchymal cells from blood into bile (Lemaitre-Coelho et al., 1978; Orlans et al., 1978). Monomeric IgA, and 11S IgA are not concentrated in bile. When dinitrophenol (DNP) is used to raise antibodies, preformed complexes of anti-DNP IgA with antigen were also found to be transported into mouse bile (Russell et al., 1981). Clearly, such a mechanism provides an ideal route for the removal of food containing immune complexes from the bloodstream, and incidentally will also re-present the antigen to the GALT of the jejunum, reinforcing the induction of normal IgA immune responses. Unfortunately this phenomenon does not occur in all species. A study performed in man has been reported in abstract (Dooley et al., 1981). [125]I- and ^{131}I-labelled dimeric and monomeric IgA were prepared. In rats, up to 32 per cent of intravenously

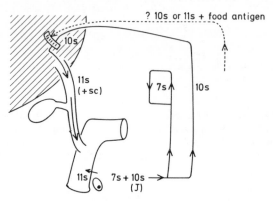

(NB only 1% of intravenously injected dimeric IgA recovered in human bile)

FIGURE 4   Relationships between IgA and the liver. 7S IgA remains in the circulation; in some species 10S IgA is removed from the blood by hepatocytes and secreted into bile as 11S IgA. Complexes of IgA and food antigen may also be removed from the blood by the liver (see text). SC, 7S 10S 11S IgA as in Figure 3.

injected dimeric IgA, but only 4 per cent of monomeric IgA, was recovered from bile after intravenous injections. In four patients, biliary recovery of dimeric IgA was less than 1 per cent. It thus seems unlikely that the liver provides an important route for removal of IgA from the serum of man, although studies with naturally occurring IgA, rather than with myeloma proteins, are awaited.

Immunoglobulins derived from the serum

In addition to locally synthesized immunoglobulins, proteins derived from the vascular and extracellular fluids make a substantial contribution to the intestinal immunoglobulin pool. There are probably a number of routes whereby plasma proteins can reach the lumen of the gut and this is more likely to occur when disease renders the mucosa 'leaky', whether or not ulceration is present. Functions, useful or otherwise, of these plasma proteins remain to be established.

IMMUNE RESPONSES TO INGESTED ANTIGEN

An antigen is defined as a substance which elicits a specific immune response when introduced into the tissues of an animal. A single protein molecule may have several antigenic determinants. Living organisms contain hundreds of different antigens and small molecules (haptens) may also act as stimulators of antibody (immunogens) when bound to a carrier protein such as serum albumin. Any antigen may evoke several types of immune response which are not mutually exclusive. In the case of antigen administered by the gut, both systemic and mucosal immune responses occur (Figure 5), and either induction or suppression of antibody- or cell-mediated immunity may be produced. It is worth emphasizing the differences between *active immunity* in which antigen-reactive cells and specific antibody develop, and *immunological tolerance* which is a specific immune resonse leading to suppression of reactions if the same antigen is subsequently given systemically. Active immune responses can readily be detected and measured in man as well as in animals, whereas the phenomenon of immunological tolerance to ingested protein has been studied mainly in small laboratory rodents.

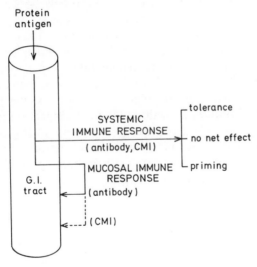

FIGURE 5　Spectrum of systemic and mucosal immune responses which may be elicited by the ingestion of a protein antigen. CMI — cell-mediated immunity.

Antigen access to the tissues

Both induction and expression of immune responses require access of antigen to the tissues of the body. Small amounts of antigen may penetrate the normal intestinal mucosa at various sites (Figure 6). In a non-immune individual,

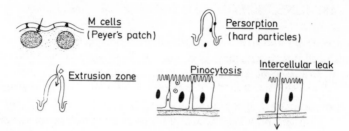

FIGURE 6   Several routes by which antigens may cross the epithelium of the small intestine.

antigen which has crossed the epithelium of the small intestine will initiate one or more patterns of immune response. In an already immunized individual, antigen access via the epithelium of the gut may lead to gastrointestinal or systemic antigen/antibody or antigen/cell interactions. However it should be emphasized that food antigens may also gain access to the circulation via the mucosa of the nose, mouth, respiratory tract, and possibly even the skin, and that even when foods have been ingested it is entirely possible that antigens gain access to normal or diseased intestinal mucosae via the bloodstream as well as by direct transport across the epithelium. It is not known whether there is increased uptake of antigen across Peyer's patches in an already immunized individual or when there is intestinal inflammation.

So far, the body of evidence is that the specialized epithelium overlying the Peyer's patches and lymphoid nodules is necessary for the presentation of antigen to the GALT and for induction of the orderly gastrointestinal immune responses (Owen, 1977). The fate of antigens which cross the mucosal barrier by other routes is uncertain, but substances which enter the tissues will be phagocytosed by macrophages in the mucosa or draining lymph nodes, or may reach the liver to be cleared by Kupffer cells.

Permeability in parasite infections

There is evidence from research in rodents that the leak of a marker molecule (horseradish peroxidase or Evan's blue) across the columnar epithelium of the small intestine is substantially increased during helminth parasite infections (Murray *et al.*, 1971; Nawa, 1979). It is likely that the worms themselves are the principal factor in producing the increase in intestinal permeability, although a contribution by IgE/mast cell mediators cannot be excluded (Ferguson and Miller, 1979). Increased permeability to a marker protein molecule, with reduction of this permeability in sodium cromoglycate-treated animals, has been documented in rats undergoing intestinal anaphylactic reactions (Byars and Ferraresi, 1976). Whether antigens crossing a permeable intestinal mucosa may be present in sufficient amount and in an appropriate immunochemical state to elicit reaginic IgE antibodies is unknown, but it is certainly true that antigens absorbed from the gut are among the wide range of materials to which allergic individuals make IgE antibodies—the immunological basis of immediate-type hypersensitivity diseases.

Permeability in IgA deficiency

It has been suggested that deficiency of IgA predisposes to food allergy because it allows increased permeability of the gut to protein and other food antigens (Taylor *et al.*, 1973). However, important experimental work relevant to this subject indicates that animals are more likely to make IgE responses when extremely small amounts of antigen are presented intermittently (Jarrett, 1977). It seems more likely that in IgA-deficient individuals there is also deficient immunoregulation and that alterations in the functions of IgE-specific suppressor T cells provide a more rational explanation for the mechanism of atopy in IgA deficiency, rather than the most simplistic hyperpermeability theories.

Systemic immune responses

Although the characteristic result of oral immunization is a local, mucosal immune response, there are a number of circumstances, especially in infants, in which active systemic immune responses develop to enteric antigens— priming for systemic immunity. Serum antibodies to cow's milk proteins are found in most normal infants and children (Ferguson, 1977b; Bahna and Heiner, 1980). In persons who have ulcerated or inflamed intestinal mucosae, and in IgA-deficient individuals, IgM and IgG class antibodies to many food proteins are to be found in the serum (Ferguson, 1976), although it is unusual for such antibodies to produce local immune reactions or to cause disease. In patients with chronic liver disease the hyperglobulinaemia is associated with high titres of serum antibodies to enteric bacteria (Triger and Wright, 1973) perhaps because the diseased liver is defective in its capacity to sequester bacterial antigens from portal blood.

Systemic immunization for IgE production to enteric antigens also occurs in atopic individuals, as discussed above, and the type of immune response, whether milk-specific IgE antibodies, or antibodies of other immunoglobulin classes, has been correlated with the amounts and duration of milk exposure in milk-allergic individuals (Firer *et al.*, 1981). By using appropriate dose schedules, circulating IgE antibodies to protein antigens can readily be induced in rats who have been fed the antigen, and there are similar critical effects of dose (Bazin and Platteau, 1976; Jarrett *et al.*, 1976).

Immunological tolerance

It has been recognized for more than half a century that the feeding of antigen may lead to a state of systemic unresponsiveness or tolerance (Wells and Osborne, 1911; Chase, 1946). Induction of systemic tolerance by feeding has been demonstrated, in experimental animals, for both limbs of the immune system, humoral and cell-mediated (Vaz *et al.*, 1977; Richman *et al.*, 1978; Mowat *et al.*, 1982).

The mechanism whereby tolerance is induced and maintained is not completely understood. Among the proposed explanations are circulating antigen–antibody complexes (André *et al.*, 1975), antigen processing by the liver (Thomas *et al.*, 1973), circulating serum factors (Kagnoff, 1980), and activation of suppressor cells in the GALT (Richman *et al.*, 1978; Ngan and Kind, 1978; Mowat and Ferguson, 1981b). It seems likely that there will be more than one suppressor or tolerogenic mechanism involved in this crucial homeostatic protective function of the gut. All food-allergic diseases including atopy can be seen as a breakdown of this protective mechanism.

Mucosal immune responses

Secretory antibodies

The immunoglobulin class, titre, and time-course of the secretory antibody responses differ substantially from serum antibody responses to enterically administered or systemic antigens. Sixty years ago Davies (1922) reported the presence of antibody in the faeces of subjects with bacterial infections, at a time when antibody was not present in the blood. The important role of IgA antibody in secretions was recognized only in the 1960s (Tomasi *et al.*, 1965) and subsequent studies in many species, with many different microbial antigens, has confirmed that a secretory antibody response involving mainly IgA, but also to a lesser extent IgM, develops within a few days of enteric immunization (Bazin, 1976; McClelland, 1979). Antibodies to foodstuffs can regularly be demonstrated in the upper intestinal secretions of children and adults (Ferguson and Carswell, 1972; Ferguson, 1976).

Mucosal cell-mediated immunity

In contrast to the secretory antibody system of the gut, mucosal cell-mediated immunity (CMI) is poorly understood, partly because techniques have only recently become available for measurement of GALT CMI. From recent experiments in mice it has become clear that certain features of intestinal pathology — crypt cell production rate and intraepithelial lymphocyte count — are reliable indicators of a delayed hypersensitivity reaction in the intestinal mucosa (Mowat and Ferguson, 1981a, 1982a), and that a leucocyte migration inhibition test, applied to mesenteric lymph nodes, also measures GALT CMI (Mowat and Ferguson, 1982b). Clinically, there is still only very indirect evidence of the presence of sensitized lymphocytes within the gut mucosa, derived from short-term organ culture studies (Ferguson *et al.*, 1975).

It seems likely that mucosal CMI responses do not occur when harmless antigens are administered to healthy individuals. However mucosal CMI can be implicated as a contributory factor in several different malabsorption syndromes (Ferguson, 1978). In patients with immunodeficiency states and malabsorption, the enteropathy may be at times due to an autoimmune process, or at other times to local immune responses to parasitic infestations such as giardiasis. Mucosal CMI to a dietary antigen is, on present evidence, the most likely cause of intestinal damage in coeliac disease, cow's milk sensitive enteropathy, and perhaps also other food allergies such as soya allergy. Local immune reactions to foods may also contribute to malabsorption in some infants with intractable diarrhoea. Clearly, in these diseases, the pathogenesis lies in the induction of CMI rather than tolerance when antigen has been fed.

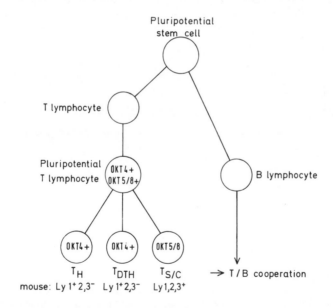

FIGURE 7 Schematic representation of T cell development from the pluripotential haematopoietic stem cell. Human cell surface markers are taken from the OKT monoclonal antibody system and the Ly classification is the equivalent for mouse lymphocytes. T_H—T helper cell; T_{DTH}—T delayed type hypersensitivity cell; $T_{S/C}$—T suppressor/cytotoxic cell. Cell surface receptors identified by monoclonal antibodies from the OKT system in man and Ly system in mice.

Critical immunoregulatory role of the T cell

T lymphocytes originate from a common pluripotential hematopoietic stem cell and their maturation is dependent in part on exposure to the environment of the thymus and in part on the presentation of antigen, for example by macrophages. T cell subclasses in peripheral blood and lymph include T helper (T_H), T suppressor cytotoxic ($T_{S/CT}$) and T delayed hypersensitivity (T_{DTH}). Although T cells were originally classified in relation to their function, these different subsets can now be recognized and identified by the presence of cell surface markers (Figure 7) (Reinherz *et al.*, 1979, 1980).

The various types of immune response which may develop after antigen is administered enterically can be explained on the basis of different patterns of stimulation of immunoregulatory T cells in the GALT (Figure 8). Within the Peyer's patches conditions are optimal for T cell interactions with antigen. The Peyer's patches contain precursors of lamina propria IgA cells, and antigen, which is presented to T cells by macrophages within the organized lymphoid tissues of the gut, leads to the induction of antigen-specific T helper cells and activation of T suppressor cells. From experiments with mouse Peyer's patch and mesenteric lymph node cells, there has been found to be dual activation of helper cells for the IgA system and suppressor cells for IgM and IgG synthesis

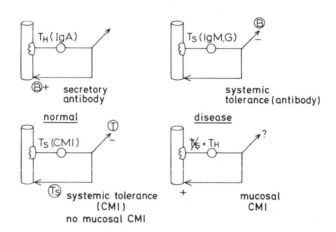

FIGURE 8   Hypothetical migration pathways of Peyer's patch T cells, after enteric administration of antigen. *Top left:* activation of antigen specific T_H IgA cells leads to stimulation of B lymphocytes which have recirculated in tandem, producing a mucosal IgA response. *Top right:* simultaneously, there is specific activation of T_S cells for IgG and IgM production leading to specific systemic tolerance. *Bottom left:* at the same time there is induction of specific T_S cells which suppress CMI responses and protect the gut from deleterious mucosal CMI reactions. *Bottom right:* in disease states, where the induction of T_S is prevented, antigen administration may lead to induction of systemic and mucosal CMI, with associated development of villous atrophy.

(Elson *et al.*, 1979; Richman *et al.*, 1981). In disease, or in experimental animals in which cyclophosphamide is used to inhibit suppressor cells, there may be stimulation of mucosal CMI (Mowat and Ferguson, 1981a). Results of these animal experiments are so consistent that they should provide an impetus for studies of immunoregulatory T cells, both in the gut and in the peripheral blood, in patients with intestinal inflammatory and allergic diseases.

INTESTINAL PERMEABILITY TO LARGE AND SMALL MOLECULES

The term 'intestinal permeability' has been applied in several different contexts.

Neonatal immunoglobulin transport

In many mammals there is active transport of proteins, particularly immuno-globulins, across the gut of the suckling infant, and this provides an important route for the transmission of passive immunity from mother to young (Brambell, 1970). Around the time of weaning there is dramatic reduction in this transmucosal protein absorption, the phenomenon of 'closure'.

Macromolecular absorption

In mammals of all ages, including human infants and adults, it has been demonstrated that when proteins are placed within the lumen of a segment of the intestine, either *in vivo* or in a gut sac *in vitro*, large molecular weight, immunogenic material crosses the wall of the gut to be detected either in blood or lymph *in vivo*, or at the serosal side of cultured intestine *in vitro*. It is not known how much of this transepithelial transport takes place across the Peyer's patch epithelium, and how much protein crosses the villus epithelium by the routes illustrated in Figure 6. In animal experiments, serum levels of antigen after oral administration are extremely variable but several groups have demonstrated a reduction in the amount of antigen absorbed across a segment of intestine if the animal has previously been orally immunized with the antigen concerned (Walker *et al.*, 1972; André *et al.*, 1974; Swarbrick *et al.*, 1979). Perhaps of relevance to food allergic reactions, intestinal uptake of macromolecules appears to be enhanced in animals infected with a helminth parasite or subjected to mild systemic or gastrointestinal anaphylaxis (Bloch *et al.*, 1979; Roberts *et al.*, 1981).

Distributed digestion

Whereas most experiments showed absorption of material of the order of 0.1–1 per cent of the administered protein, Hemmings and his colleagues have reported that much greater amounts of dietary proteins cross the gut mucosa in the form of large molecules. In a study of adult rats they reported that up to 40 per cent of a dose of bovine gamma globulin was absorbed as large molecular weight material, typically in the range of 20,000–50,000 Daltons. They claimed that tissue cells throughout the body were loaded with much foreign protein of dietary origin, the fate of which was to be degraded over a protracted period. They coined the term 'distributed digestion' and suggested that this occurred in all body cells rather than in the gut lumen (Hemmings and Williams, 1978). These surprising findings have not been confirmed by other workers, and it seems likely that their observations were due to small radio-labelled fragments of exogenous protein which bound to native proteins after absorption, thus mimicking the uptake of macromolecules (Udall *et al.*, 1981).

Persorption

Another phenomenon, which may or may not lead to induction of immuno-logical responses to fed proteins, is that of persorption—the transportation of solid particles of foods and other substances through or between the intestinal epithelial cells (Volkheimer and Schultz, 1968; Le Févre and Joél, 1977).

Passive penetration of small molecules

In contrast to the above, immunologically relevant, uses of the term permeability, many physiologists study the transport of much smaller molecules. The columnar epithelial cells of the small intestine are held together firmly at the luminal surface by junctional complexes. Many substances, including ions and various nutrients, may be actively transported across the brush border of the cells and there is also a route which allows passive penetration of water, ions, and other small molecules such as sugars. This latter is via hypothetical water-filled pores, perhaps by a paracellular pathway through the tight junctions (Frömter and Diamond, 1972). Diffusion of small molecules such as tritiated water or xylose across the small intestinal epithelium is inversely related to molecular size (Fordtran *et al.*, 1967). Larger molecules such as dextran of radius 1.25 nm will also pass through small bowel mucosa but the number of large pores, admitting these larger molecules, seems to be lower than the number of small pores (Wheeler *et al.*, 1978). It is not known whether large complex molecules such as food proteins also pass through these large pores, or whether they pass by one or more other routes.

Clinical studies of intestinal permeability

Tests for measurement of permeability of the human intestine to molecules such as marker sugars or dextrans have been developed, and the results indicate substantially increased permeability of the mucosa to larger probe molecules in patients with coeliac disease (Menzies *et al.*, 1979; Cobden *et al.*, 1980). Increased permeability to a large probe molecule was also found in some patients with atopic eczema (Jackson *et al.*, 1981). Studies which combine permeability to marker molecules and to protein antigens should now be pursued, both in experimental animals and in man.

Clinical investigation of protein antigen absorption across the gastro-intestinal tract has been applied in healthy individuals, and in patients with atopic diseases and food allergic states. Intestinal absorption of immuno-reactive protein by normal infants and children was well documented in the 1920s (Anderson *et al.*, 1925; Sussman *et al.*, 1928). These early studies relied on biological phenomena such as passive cutaneous anaphylaxis to demonstrate the presence of antigens in serum. Techniques such as radio-immunoassay now allow detection of food protein antigens in human serum with remarkable sensitivity. In one recent study, beta-lactoglobulin was detected in the sera of three normal individuals shortly after drinking milk, at concentrations of 0.1–3 ng per ml (Paganelli and Levinsky, 1980). In a study of children, many of whom suffered from malabsorption, the egg protein ovalbumin was detected in the serum of 34 of 42 children, with peak concen-trations 2 hours after ingestion of eggs (Danneus *et al.*, 1979). Sodium cromoglycate treatment of these children not only produced beneficial effects on egg-related symptoms, but also decreased serum concentrations of ovalbumin after egg feeding in sodium cromoglycate-treated patients. It is not yet established how this anti-allergic drug acts to reduce absorption of antigens.

Circulating immune complexes

Since most normal individuals have low titres of circulating antibody to food proteins, it is not surprising that sensitive techniques have revealed the presence of circulating immune complexes shortly after ingestion of foodstuffs both in healthy and in food-allergic subjects (Paganelli *et al.*, 1979, 1981). Specific IgE-containing complexes have been reported in two egg-allergic patients, after oral challenge with the food allergen (Brostoff *et al.*, 1979a). In these patients, and in some of the previously studied subjects with other types of immune complexes in the circulation after feeding, pretreatment with oral sodium cromoglycate relieved symptoms and reduced the amounts of circulating immune complexes. Levinsky has shown that the immunoglobulin in food-related immune complexes in normal subjects is predominantly IgA (Levinsky *et al.*, 1981), whereas in food-allergic subjects the complexes may also contain IgG and IgE, and may bind component (Brostoff *et al.*, 1979a,b). This again highlights the potential role of defective immunoregulation as the underlying mechanism of food-allergic states. Normal immune responses, with high titres of anti-food IgA antibodies, will lead to the production of harmless complexes which are rapidly cleared, whereas if there have been aberrant immune responses to fed antigen, further ingestion of the foodstuff leads to the formation of immune complexes in which all immunoglobulin classes may be involved. Complex interactions of different facets of the inflammatory response may thus be elicited—for example complement fixing, antigen-excess immune complexes may be localized in skin and lungs by the triggering of antigen-specific IgE sensitized mast cells to release mediators of vascular permeability. With complement activation, chemotactic factors are released to attract neutrophils and mononuclear phagocytes which accentuate the inflammatory response by the release of proteolytic enzymes (Levinsky et al., 1981).

EFFECTS OF LOCAL IMMUNE REACTIONS ON GASTROINTESTINAL STRUCTURE AND FUNCTION

There is a substantial body of evidence that abnormal immunological reactions in the gastrointestinal tract alter its structure and function and thereby cause or contribute to disease processes. Several clearly documented food-allergic diseases are discussed in other chapters of this book and will not be considered further in this section. However it is appropriate to highlight several points of general principle with regard to intestinal mucosal histology and functional bowel disorders.

Mucosal hypersensitivity reactions

An immune reaction may cause tissue damage or disease, either as an unavoidable side-effect of a protective function, or as a primary pathological event. The term hypersensitivity is often used to describe this process, as a state of the previously immunized animal or person in which tissue damage results from the immune reaction to a further dose of antigen. Hypersensitivity may be antibody-mediated or cell-mediated, and each reaction is triggered by one or more of a range of immunological components. The tissue damage is mediated either by soluble factors, by activated polymorphonuclear leucocytes or macrophages, or by direct membrane effects between the immune cell and antigen on the membrane of another cell. The various types of hypersensitivity are not mutually exclusive, and since the time-course of their development varies according to the type and to the antigen concerned, they may occur all at once or in sequence.

The effects of humoral and cell-mediated immune reactions on the histopathological appearances of intestinal mucosa have been studied both for the small intestinal mucosa and also the colon. The observations have been made mainly in experimental animals, although there is limited clinical information to back up this animal work. Full details, including references, have been published elsewhere (Ferguson and Mowat, 1980; Ferguson, 1981a; Earnshaw *et al.*, 1982). The general features of intestinal histopathology which occur in reaginic, immune complex and T cell-mediated hypersensitivity reactions are summarized in Figure 9.

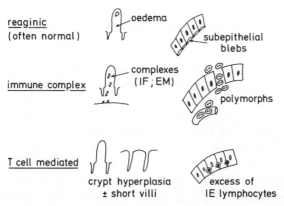

FIGURE 9   Histopathological changes in experimental hypersensitivity of the small bowel. IF—immunofluorescence; EM—electron microscopy.

Reaginic hypersensitivity

In general, this does not produce any change in intestinal histopathology and earlier reports of degranulation of mast cells have not been confirmed. There is, however, increased permeability to large molecules (see above) and it is likely that the inflammation associated with this type of reaction creates appropriate conditions for further development of other types of hypersensitivity involving antigen–antibody complexes and cells.

Immune complex hypersensitivity

This has been induced both by instilling antigen into the lumen of a segment of gut, and by intravenous injection of immune complexes. In general, this leads to infiltration of the tissues with polymorphonuclear leucocytes and deposition of immune complexes, without substantial alterations in general mucosal architecture.

T cell-mediated hypersensitivity

This has been shown in several different animal models to produce stimulation of mitosis in the crypts of Lieberkühn—as an enteropathic effect. It is possible that it achieves this by affecting adhesion of enterocytes to one another and to the basement membrane, and by recruitment and activation of lymphoid cells in the mucosa. As discussed above, local cell-mediated immune reactions probably contribute to the intestinal pathology and malabsorption in several chronic malabsorption syndromes, including coeliac disease and cow's milk protein-sensitive enteropathy.

Clinical methods for investigation of intestinal hypersensitivity

Clinical studies of GALT immunity have generally concerned the cells in mucosal biopsies. By comparing biopsies taken at different times, it is possible to obtain limited information on the dynamics of mucosal changes during adverse reactions, for example in food-related immune responses. In particular, serial studies of intestinal mucosa (permeability, morphology, etc.) performed after antigen challenge or in the weeks after initiation of dietary or pharmacological treatment, may provide useful information. If immediate hypersensitivity is present, there may be some oedema or eosinophil infiltrate in biopsies taken shortly after antigen challenge, and the patient may of course develop anaphylactic reactions, skin rash, or wheeze. If immune complex-mediated mechanisms are suspected, complexes may be found in the tissues, there may be polymorphonuclear infiltrate and systemic manifestations such as fever and abdominal pain, a drop in serum complement levels, and an appearance of serum immune complexes may occur. Evidence of local cell-mediated mechanisms is more difficult to obtain but may be inferred from the development of histological changes such as a flat mucosa with lymphocyte infiltration, 1–2 days after antigen challenge.

Gastrointestinal motility

Normal gastrointestinal motility is essential to all of the other functions of the gut, and deviations from normal of motility, or abnormal perception of a normal pattern of motility, can produce a wide range of symptoms referrable to the gastrointestinal tract and often related to foods. The function of the oesophagus is simply to propel food from the mouth to the stomach but a competent lower oesophageal sphincter is necessary to prevent reflux of gastric contents back into the oesophagus. The regular contractions of the gastric antrum steadily supply partially digested foods to the small intestine, within which there is segmentation as well as onward propulsion of secretions by peristalsis. The volume and physicochemical nature of the contents of the small intestine vary considerably, and very large amounts of water and electrolytes are secreted and absorbed across the mucosa, even in the normal individual. Within the colon, bacterial metabolism, particularly in the caecum, leads to gas production and after a slow transit through the distal colon, faeces are partially dried and stored, so that the frequency of defaecation may be controlled.

Several experimental and clinical observations have unequivocally shown that local immunological reactions influence gastrointestinal motility. Local immediate hypersensitivity reactions have been produced by transfer of reagin-containing serum into the small or large bowel mucosa, followed a few days later by exposure to antigen (Gray et al., 1940; Gray and Walzer, 1938; Walzer et al., 1938). This treatment led to prepyloric or pyloric spasm, hyperperistalsis of the small and large intestines, oedema with mucus secretion, and in the rectum, tenesmus. Of course, among the many fully documented and clear-cut acute reactions to ingestion of a foodstuff to which a patient is allergic, are nausea, vomiting, abdominal pain, and diarrhoea. Some of the symptoms of the so-called 'specific adaptive syndrome' (Mackarness, 1976) are gastrointestinal, and are reminiscent of those which have been evoked by food-allergic reactions in sensitized individuals. Nevertheless there is need for great caution in extrapolating results from known food-allergic individuals to the many members of the general population whose symptoms indicate altered gastrointestinal motility. In most causes these symptoms are due to the irritable bowel syndrome, a condition for which there is no evidence of an allergic basis.

Prevalence of the irritable bowel syndrome

The irritable bowel syndrome was first recognized as a symptom complex in patients presenting to gastroenterologists with abdominal pain and/or a change in bowel habit. However with further clinical experience it is clear that such patients may have symptoms to indicate abnormal motility of any part of the gastrointestinal tract — for example globus, heartburn, nausea, upper abdominal pain without ulceration, colicky central abdominal pain, colonic pain, bloating, diarrhoea, or constipation. We found that one-third of patients presenting at our specialist gastrointestinal clinic ultimately had a diagnosis of irritable bowel syndrome made (Ferguson et al., 1977).

Recently it has been found that symptoms of abnormal intestinal motility, identical to those of the irritable bowel syndrome, are frequently present in apparently healthy people. Four clinically distinct functional bowel syndromes were found to exist in almost one-third of the 301 healthy British subjects studied by Thompson and Heaton (1980). Abdominal pain, a feeling of incomplete evacuation after defaecation, urgency, scybala, runny stools, straining at stool, borborygmi, distension, heartburn, and laxative use were all very common. The typical symptom pattern of the spastic irritable bowel syndrome occurred in 13.6 per cent of subjects; 7 per cent suffered non-colonic pain that was commonly associated with heartburn; a further 3.7 per cent had painless diarrhoea; and 6 per cent suffered painless constipation. Most of these subjects had not consulted a doctor. Clearly factors other than the mere existence of these intestinal motility disorder symptoms lead to a patient's decision to consult a general practitioner and to the general practitioner's decision to seek confirmation of the diagnosis of motility disorder by requesting a hospital consultation.

The symptoms of lactose intolerance, in lactase-deficient individuals, are rather similar to those of the irritable bowel syndrome (Ferguson, 1981b). In a recent study, we asked multi-racial groups of apparently healthy doctors attending postgraduate courses to make a self-diagnosis of the irritable bowel syndrome and we also enquired of symptoms of lactose intolerance (Fowkes and Ferguson, 1980). We found that 13 per cent of white doctors and 18 per cent of non-white doctors thought that they had the irritable bowel syndrome, and the prevalence of cow's milk intolerance in non-white doctors with the irritable bowel syndrome was much higher than in their counterparts who had no such symptoms. These results suggested that motility disorders of the intestine may in some cases be a manifestation of lactase deficiency, although this is unusual in white, British-born adults.

Gastrointestinal gas

Some patients who think they have food allergy complain of eructation of gas, abdominal bloating, and increased passage of flatus. Although there is no evidence that immunological reactions influence intestinal gas production or transit in any way, it is appropriate to finish this chapter with a brief account of recent research on the subject of gastrointestinal gas (well reviewed by Levitt and Bond, 1980). The normal intestinal content of gas is of the order of 100–200 ml and in a careful study of 12 patients who complained of excessive gas, abdominal pain and bloating, there were no differences from controls in the composition of or the accumulation rate of intestinal gas (Lasser *et al.*, 1975). However there was evidence of abnormal intestinal motility in that the patients who complained of severe pain during the study had a longer intestinal transit time of gas than controls (40 versus 22 minutes). Thus disordered intestinal motility in combination with an abnormal pain response to gut distension, rather than increased volume of gut gas, was thought to lead to this group of symptoms in these patients.

The amount of gas passed per rectum varies considerably from individual to individual, ranging from 200 to 2000 ml per day, with a mean of around 600. This gas is produced by bacterial fermentation of various substrates which have not been absorbed by the small intestine. Thus dramatic alterations in the diet — for example increased milk intake in a lactase-deficient individual, or a diet rich in beans or wheat in a normal individual, substantially increase gas production and gas expulsion rate (Levitt *et al.*, 1976; Steggerda, 1968; Anderson *et al.*, 1981). Alterations in the colonic flora may also lead to increased gas production, because colonic bacteria not only produce but also metabolize hydrogen and other gases, so that changed bacterial flora is the likely explanation of the relatively frequent though transient colonic symptoms in patients who have received broad-spectrum antibiotics.

As with virtually all facets of the physiology of the digestive system, the nature of foods consumed will of course lead to variations in sensations associated with digestion, and in the nature and amount of the undigested faecal residue. It must be emphasized that discomfort and awareness of various aspects of digestion are frequently found in healthy individuals, and a standard, relatively high residue and varied diet should be recommended for patients with gastrointestinal motility disorders.

REFERENCES

Anderson, A. F., Scloss, D. M., and Myers, C. (1925). The intestinal absorption of antigenic protein by normal infants *Proc. Soc. Exp. Biol. Med.*, **23**, 180-2.

Anderson, I. H., Levine, A. S., and Levitt, M. D. (1981). Incomplete absorption of the carbohydrate in all-purpose wheat flour *N. Engl. J. Med.*, **304**, 891-2.

André, C., Heremans, J. F., Vaerman, J., and Cambiaso, C. L. (1975). A mechanism for the induction of immunological tolerance by antigen feeding: antigen-antibody complexes. *J. Exp. Med.*, **142**, 1509-19.

André, C., Lambert, R., Bazin, H., and Heremans, J. F. (1974). Interference of oral immunization with the intestinal absorption of heterologous albumin. *Eur. J. Immunol.*, **4**, 701-4.

Bahna, S. L., and Heiner, D. C. (1980). *Allergy to Milk*. Grune and Stratton, New York, pp.23-44.

Bazin, H. (1976). The secretory antibody system. In: *Immunological Aspects of the Liver and Gastrointestinal Tract* (eds Anne Ferguson and R. N. M. MacSween), pp.33-82. MTP Press, Lancaster.

Bazin, H., and Platteau, B. (1976). Production of circulating reaginic (IgE) antibodies by oral administration of ovalbumin to rats. *Immunology*, **30**, 679-84.

Bloch, K. J., Bloch, D. B., Stearns, M., and Walker, W. A. (1979). Intestinal uptake of macromolecules. VI. Uptake of protein antigen *in vivo* in normal rats and in rats infected with *Nippostrongylus brasiliensis* or subjected to milk systemic anaphylaxis. *Gastroenterology*, **77**, 1039-44.

Brambell, F. W. R. (1970). The transmission of passive immunity from mother to young. In: *Frontiers of Biology, No. 18*. North Holland, Amsterdam.

Brandtzaeg, P., and Baklien, K. (1976). Immunohistochemical studies on the formation and epithelial transport of immunoglobulins in normal and diseased human intestinal mucosa. *Scand. J. Gastroenterol.*, **11**, 1-45.

Brostoff, J., Carini, C., Wraith, D. G., and Johns, P. (1979a). Production of IgE complexes by allergen challenge in atopic patients and the effect of sodium cromoglycate. *Lancet*, **1**, 1268-70.

Brostoff, J., Carini, C., Wraith, D. C., Paganelli, R., and Levinsky, R. J. (1979b). Immune complexes in atopy. In: *The Mast Cell* (eds J. Pepys and A. M. Edwards), pp.380-93. Pitman, London.

Byars, N. E., and Ferraresi, R. W. (1976). Intestinal anaphylaxis in the rat as a model of food allergy. *Clin. Exp. Immunol.*, **24**, 352-6.

Chase, M. W. (1946). Inhibition of experimental drug allergy by prior feeding of the sensitizing agent. *Proc. Soc. Exp. Biol. Med.*, **61**, 257–9.

Cobden, I., Rothwell, J., and Axon, A. T. R. (1980). Intestinal permeability and screening tests for coeliac disease. *Gut*, **21**, 512–18.

Dannaeus, A., Inganäs, M., Johansson, S. G. O., and Foucard, T. (1979). Intestinal uptake of ovalbumin in malabsorption and food allergy in relation to serum IgG antibody and orally administered sodium cromoglycate. *Clin. Allergy.*, **9**, 263–70.

Davies, A. (1922). Investigation into the serological properties of dysentery stools. *Lancet*, **2**, 1009–12.

Dooley, J. S., Potter, B. J., Thomas, H. C., and Sherlock, S. (1981). Comparative study of biliary secretion of labelled human dimeric and monomeric IgA in rats and in man. *Gut*, **22**, A872.

Earnshaw, P., Busuttil, A., and Ferguson, A. (1982). Relevance of colonic mucosal inflammation to the aetiology of colorectal cancer. In: *Recent Results in Cancer Research*, No. 83 (ed. W. Duncan), pp. 31–400. Springer-Verlag, Heidelberg.

Elson, C. O., Heck, J. A., and Strober, W. (1979). T-cell regulation of murine IgA-synthesis *J. Exp. Med.*, **149**, 632–43.

Ferguson, A. (1976). Coeliac disease and gastrointestinal food allergy. In: *Immunological Aspects of the Liver and Gastrointestinal Tract* (eds Anne Ferguson and R. N. M. MacSween), pp.153–202. MTP Press, Lancaster.

Ferguson, A. (1977a). Intraepithelial lymphocytes of the small intestine. *Gut*, **18**, 921–37.

Ferguson, A. (1977b). Immunogenicity of cows' milk in man. *La Ricerca*, **7**, 211–19.

Ferguson, A. (1978). Lymphocytes and cell mediated immunity in the small intestine. In: *Advanced Medicine* (ed. D. Weatherall), pp.278–93. Pitman Medical, Tunbridge Wells.

Ferguson, A. (1981a). Chronic diarrhoeal disease in older children. In: *Recent Advances in Paediatrics* (ed. D. Hull), pp.97–136. Churchill Livingstone, London.

Ferguson, A. (1981b). Diagnosis and treatment of lactose intolerance. *Br. Med. J.*, **283**, 1423–4.

Ferguson, A., and Carswell, F. (1972). Precipitins to dietary proteins in the serum and upper intestinal secretions of coeliac children. *Br. Med. J.*, **1**, 75–7.

Ferguson, A., and Miller, H. R. P. (1979). Role of the mast cell in the defence against gut parasites. In: *The Mast Cell* (eds. J. Pepys and A. N. Edwards), pp.159–65. Pitman, London.

Ferguson, A., and Mowat, A. Mc.I. (1980). Immunological mechanisms in the small intestine. In: *Recent Advances in Gastrointestinal Pathology* (ed. R. Wright), pp.93–103. W. B. Saunders, Eastbourne.

Ferguson, A., MacDonald, T. T., McClure, J. P., and Holden, R. J. (1975). Cell-mediated immunity to gliadin within the small intestinal mucosa in coeliac disease. *Lancet*, **1**, 895–7.

Ferguson, A., Sircus, W., and Eastwood, M. A. (1977). Frequency of 'Functional' gastrointestinal disorders. *Lancet*, **1**, 613–14 (letter).

Firer, M. A., Hosking, C. S., and Hill, D. J. (1981). Effect of antigen load on development of milk antibodies in infants allergic to milk. *Br. Med. J.*, **283**, 693–6.

Fordtran, J. S., Rector, F. C., Locklear, T. W., and Ewton, M. F. (1967). Water and solute movement in the small intestine of patients with sprue *J. Clin. Invest.*, **46**, 287–98.

Fowkes, G., and Ferguson, A. (1980). Prevalence of self-diagnosed irritable bowel syndrome and cows' milk intolerance in white and non-white doctors. *Scott. Med. J.*, **26**, 41–4.

Frömter, E., and Diamond, J. (1972). Route of passive ion permeation in epithelia. *Nature; New Biol.*, **235**, 9–13.

Gray, I., Harten, M., and Walzer, M. (1940). Studies in mucous membrane hypersensitiveness. IV. The allergic reaction in the passively sensitised mucous membranes of the ileum and colon in humans *Ann. Int. Med.*, **13**, 2050–6.

Gray, I., and Walzer, M. (1938). Studies in mucous membrane hypersensitiveness. III. The allergic reaction of the passively sensitised rectal mucous membrane. *Am. J. Dig. Dis. Nutr.*, **4**, 707–12.

Guy-Grand, D., Griscelli, C., and Vassali, P. (1978). The mouse gut T-lymphocyte, a novel type of T cell: nature, origin and traffic in normal and graft-versus-host conditions. *J. Exp. Med.*, **148**, 1661–77.

Hemmings, W. A., and Williams, E. W. (1978). Transport of large breakdown products of dietary protein through the gut wall. *Gut*, **19**, 715–23.

Husband, A. J., and Gowans, J. L. (1978). The origin and antigen-dependent distribution of IgA-containing cells in the intestine. *J. Exp. Med.*, **148**, 1146–60.

Jackson, P. G., Lessof, M. H., Baker, R. W. R., Ferrett, J., and MacDonald, D. M. (1981). Intestinal permeability in patients with eczema and food allergy. *Lancet*, **1**, 1285–6.

Jarrett, E. E. E. (1977). Activation of IgE regulatory mechanisms by transmucosal absorption of antigen. *Lancet*, **2**, 223–5.

Jarrett, E. E. E., Haig, D. M., McDougall, W., and McNulty, E. (1976). Rat IgE production. II. Primary and booster reaginic antibody responses following intradermal or oral immunisation. *Immunology*, **30**, 671–8.

Kagnoff, M. F. (1980). Effects of antigen feeding on intestinal and systemic immune responses. IV. Similarity between the suppressor factor in mice after erythrocyte-lysate injection and erythrocyte feeding. *Gastroenterology*, **79**, 54–61.

Lasser, R. B., Bond, J. H., and Levitt, M. D. (1975). The role of intestinal gas in functional abdominal pain. *N. Engl. J. Med.*, **293**, 524–6.

Le Févre, M. E., and Joél, D. D. (1977). Intestinal absorption of particulate matter. *Life Sciences*, **21**, 1403–8.

Lemaitre-Coelho, I., Jackson, G. D. F., and Vaerman, J. P. (1978). High levels of secretory IgA and free secretory component in the serum of rats with bile duct obstruction. *J. Exp. Med.*, **147**, 934–9.

Levinsky, R. J., Paganelli, R., Robertson, D. M., and Atherton, D. J. (1981). Handling of food antigens and their complexes by normal and allergic individuals. In: *The Immunology of Infant Feeding* (ed. A. W. Wilkinson), pp.23–30. Plenum Press, New York.

Levitt, M. D., and Bond, J. H. (1980). Intestinal gas. In: *Scientific Foundations of Gastroenterology* (eds. W. Sircus and A. N. Smith), pp.492–8. Heinemann, London.

Levitt, M. D., Lasser, R. B., Schwartz, J. S., and Bond, J. H. (1976). Studies of a flatulent patient. *N. Engl. J. Med.*, **295**, 260–2.

Mackarness, R. (1976). *Not All In The Mind*. Pan, London.

Mayrhofer, G. (1977). Sites of synthesis and localisation of IgE in rats infected with *Nippostrongylus brasiliensis*. In *Ciba Foundation Symposium*, No. 46, pp.155–75.

McClelland, D. B. L. (1979). Bacterial and viral infections of the gastrointestinal tract. In: *Immunology of the Gastrointestinal Tract* (ed. P. Asquith), pp.214–45. Churchill Livingstone, Edinburgh.

Menzies, I. S., Laker, M. F., Pounder, R., Bull, J., Heyer, S., Wheeler, P. G., and Creamer, B. (1979). Abnormal intestinal permeability to sugars in villous atrophy. *Lancet*, **2**, 1107–9.

Mowat, A. McI., and Ferguson, A. (1981a). Hypersensitivity reactions in the small intestine. 5. Induction of cell mediated immunity to a dietary antigen. *Clin. Exp. Immunol.*, **43**, 574–82.

Mowat, A. McI., and Ferguson, A. (1981b). Hypersensitivity reactions in the small intestine. 6. Pathogenesis of the graft-versus-host reaction in the small intestinal mucosa. *Transplantation*, **32**, 238–43.

Mowat, A. McI., and Ferguson, A. (1982a). Intraepithelial lymphocyte count and crypt hyperplasia measure the mucosal component of the graft-versus-host reaction in mouse small intestine. *Gastroenterology*. (In press.)

Mowat, A. McI., and Ferguson, A. (1982b). Migration inhibition of lymph node lymphocytes as an assay for regional cell mediated immunity in the intestinal lymphoid tissues of mice immunised orally with ovalbumin. *Immunology* (submitted).

Mowat, A. McI., Strobel, S., Drummond, H. E., and Ferguson, A. (1982). Immunological responses to fed protein antigens in mice. 1. Reversal of oral tolerance to ovalbumin by cyclophosphamide. *Immunology*, **45**, 105–13.

Murray, M., Jarrett, W. F., and Jennings, F. W. (1971). Mast cells and macromolecular leak in intestinal immunological reactions. The influence of sex of rats infected with *Nippostrongylus brasiliensis*. *Immunology*, **21**, 17–31.

Nawa, Y. (1979). Increased permeability of gut mucosa in rats infected with *Nippostrongylus brasiliensis*. *Int. J. Parasitol.*, **9**, 251–5.

Ngan, J., and Kind, L. S. (1978). Suppressor T-cells for IgE and IgG in Peyer's patches of mice made tolerant by the oral administration of ovalbumin. *J. Immunol.*, **120**, 861–5.

Orlans, E., Peppard, J., Reynolds, J., and Hall, J. (1978). Rapid active transport of immunoglobulin A from blood to bile. *J. Exp. Med.*, **147**, 588–92.

Owen, R. L. (1977). Sequential uptake of horseradish peroxidase by lymphoid follicle epithelium of Peyer's patches in the normal unobstructed mouse intestine: an ultrastructural study. *Gastroenterology*, **72**, 440–51.

Owen, R. L., and Jones, A. L. (1974). Epithelial cell specialization within human Peyer's patches: an ultrastructural study of intestinal lymphoid follicles. *Gastroenterology*, **66**, 189–203.

Oxelius, V. A., Laurell, A. B., Lindquist, B., Golebiowska, H., Axelsson, U., Björkander, J., and Hanson, L. A. (1981). IgG subclasses in selective IgA deficiency: importance of IgG_2–IgA deficiency. *N. Engl. J. Med.*, **304**, 1476–7.

Paganelli, R., and Levinsky, R. J. (1980). Solid phase radioimmunoassay for detection of circulating food protein antigens in human serum. *J. Immunol. Methods*, **37**, 333–41.

Paganelli, R., Levinsky, R. J., Brostoff, J., and Wraith, D. G. (1979). Immune complexes containing food proteins in normal and atopic subjects after oral challenge and effect of sodium cromoglycate on antigen absorption. *Lancet*, **1**, 1270–2.

Paganelli, R., Levinsky, R. J., and Atherton, D. J. (1981). Detection of specific antigen within circulating immune complexes: validation of the assay and its application to food antigen–antibody complexes formed in healthy and food allergic subjects. *Clin. Exp. Immunol.*, **46**, 44–53.

Parrott, D. M. V. (1976). The gut-associated lymphoid tissues and gastrointestinal immunity. In: *Immunological Aspects of the Liver and Gastrointestinal Tract* (eds A. Ferguson and R. N. M. MacSween), pp.1–32. MTP Press, Lancaster.

Parrott, D. M. V., and Ferguson, A. (1974). Selective migration of lymphocytes within the mouse small intestine. *Immunology*, **26**, 571–88.

Reinherz, E. L, Kung, P. C., Goldstein, G., and Schlossman, S. F. (1979). Separation of functional subsets of human T cells by a monoclonal antibody. *Proc. Natl. Acad. Sci. U.S.A.*, **76**, 4061-5.

Reinherz, E. L., Kung, P. C., Goldstein, G., and Schlossman, S. F. (1980). A monoclonal antibody reaction with the human cytotoxic/suppressor T cell subset previously defined by a heteroantiserum termed TH2. *J. Immunol.*, **124**, 1301-7.

Richman, L. K., Chiller, J. M., Brown, W. R., Hanson, D. G., and Van, N. M. (1978). Enterically induced immunologic tolerance. I. Induction of suppressor T-lymphocytes by intragastric administration of soluble proteins. *J. Immunol.*, **121**, 2429-34.

Richman, L. K., Graeff, A. S., Yarchoan, R., and Strober, W. (1981). Simultaneous induction of antigen-specific IgA helper T cells and IgG suppressor T cells in the murine Peyer's patch after protein feeding. *J. Immunol.*, **126**, 2079-83.

Roberts, S. A., Reinhardt, M. C., Paganelli, R., and Levinsky, R. J. (1981). Specific antigen exclusion and non-specific facilitation of antigen entry across the gut in rats allergic to food proteins. *Clin. Exp. Immunol.*, **45**, 131-6.

Rosekrans, P. C. M., Meijer, C. J. L. M., Van der Wal, A. M., and Lindeman, J. (1980a). Allergic proctitis, a clinical and immunopathological entity. *Gut*, **21**, 1017-23.

Rosekrans, P. C. M., Meijer, C. J. L. M., Cornelisse, C. J., Van der Wal, A. M., and Lindeman, J. (1980b). Use of morphometry and immunohistochemistry of small intestinal biopsy specimens in the diagnosis of food allergy. *J. Clin. Pathol.*, **33**, 125-30.

Russell, M. W., Brown, T. A., and Mestecky, J. (1981). Role of serum IgA: hepatobiliary transport of circulating antigen. *J. Exp. Med.*, **153**, 968-76.

Selby, W. S., Janossy, G., Goldstein, G., and Jewell, D. P. (1981a). T lymphocyte subsets in human intestinal mucosa. *Clin. Exp. Immunol.*, **44**, 453-8.

Selby, W. S., Janossy, G., and Jewell, D. P. (1981b). Immunohistological characterisation of intraepithelial lymphocytes of the human gastrointestinal tract. *Gut*, **22**, 169-76.

Steggerda, F. R. (1968). Gastrointestinal gas following food consumption. *Ann. N. Y. Acad. Sci.*, **150**, 57-66.

Stokes, C. R., Soothill, J. F., and Turner, M. W. (1975). Immune exclusion is a function of IgA. *Nature*, **255**, 745-6.

Strobel, S., Miller, H. R. P., and Ferguson, A. (1981). Human intestinal mucosal mast cells. Evaluation of fixation and staining techniques. *J. Clin. Pathol.*, **34**, 851-8.

Sussman, H., Davidson, A., and Walzer, M. (1928). Absorption of undigested proteins in human beings. *Arch. Int. Med.*, **42**, 409-14.

Swarbrick, E. T., Stokes, C. R., and Soothill, J. F. (1979). Absorption of antigens after oral immunisation and the simultaneous induction of specific systemic tolerance. *Gut*, **20**, 121-5.

Taylor, B., Norman, A. P., Orgel, H. A., Stokes, C. R., Turner, M. W., and Soothill, J. F. (1973). Transient IgA deficiency and pathogenesis of infantile atopy. *Lancet*, **2**, 111-3.

Thomas, H. C., MacSween, R. N. M., and White, R. G. (1973). Role of the liver in controlling the immunogenicity of commensal bacteria in the gut. *Lancet*, **1**, 1288-91.

Thompson, W. G., and Heaton, K. W. (1980). Functional bowel disorders in apparently healthy people. *Gastroenterology*, **79**, 283-8.

Tomasi, T. B., Tan, E. M., Solomon, A., and Prendergast, R. A. (1965). Characteristics of an immune system common to certain external secretions. *J. Exp. Med.*, **121**, 101-24.

Triger, D. R., and Wright, R. (1973). Hyperglobulinaemia in liver disease. *Lancet*, **1**, 1494-6.

Udall, J. N., Bloch, K. J., Fritze, L., and Walker, W. A. (1981). Binding of exogenous protein fragments to native proteins: possible explanation for the over estimations of uptake of extrinsically labelled macromolecules from the gut. *Immunology*, **42**, 251–7.

Vaz, N. M., Maia, L. C. S., Hanson, D. G., and Lynch, J. M. (1977). Inhibition of homocytotropic antibody responses in adult inbred mice by previous feeding of the specific antigen. *J. Allergy Clin. Immunol.*, **60**, 110–15.

Volkheimer, G., and Schulz, F. H. (1968). The phenomenon of persorption. *Digestion*, **1**, 213–18.

Walker, W. A., and Isselbacher, K. J. (1977). Intestinal antibodies. *N. Engl. J. Med.*, **297**, 767–73.

Walker, W. A., Isselbacher, K. J., and Bloch, K. J. (1972). Intestinal uptake of macromolecules: effect of oral immunisation. *Science*, **177**, 608–10.

Walzer, M., Gray, J., Straus, H. W., and Livingstone, S. (1938). Studies in experimental hypersensitiveness in the rhesus monkey. IV. The allergic reaction in passively locally sensitized abdominal organs. *J. Immunol.*, **34**, 91–5.

Wells, H. G., and Osborne, T. B. (1911). The biological reaction against vegetable proteins. I. Anaphylaxis. *J. Infect. Dis.*, **8**, 66–124.

Wheeler, P. G., Menzies, I. S., and Creamer, B. (1978). Effect of hyperosmolar stimuli and coeliac disease on the permeability of the human gastrointestinal tract. *Clin. Sci. Mol. Med.*, **54**, 495–501.

Clincal Reactions to Food
Edited by M. H. Lessof
© 1983 John Wiley & Sons Ltd.

Food Allergy in Childhood

J. F. Soothill

*Department of Immunology,
Institute of Child Health, London*

FOOD INTOLERANCE IN CHILDHOOD

Despite the excellent clinical investigations of Prausnitz, who transferred immediate sensitivity from his fish-sensitive friend Küstner to his own skin as long ago as 1921, food allergy has been irrationally questioned, and under-diagnosed, especially in children. Most families with children who get angioedema or urticaria quickly after taking a single food (e.g. strawberries) recognize it quickly and successfully treat the child. The medical contribution to such a process is often small, unless the child develops respiratory obstruction or anaphylaxis—important medical emergencies. In contrast to this, many food allergies (e.g. eczema) are slow to come on, and the child is often allergic to many foods, so that the cause-and-effect relationship with food is often impossible for the parent to observe and is frequently missed by the non-specialist medical observer. One food allergy of childhood, coeliac disease, was observed early—by luck and astuteness—by Dicke. The discovery of the associated intestinal biopsy lesion of subtotal villous atrophy has helped in achieving its general acceptance, but not all wheat allergy is associated with this lesion, and at least partial villous atrophy may be associated with allergy to other foods. The acceptance of other food allergies has been delayed by the lack of appropriate diagnostic tests; but the clear-cut importance of food allergy in many disease processes, and the obvious complexity of diagnosis in many, should undermine the widespread and misplaced scepticism in this field. However, many more systematic controlled studies are needed before the full scope is established, and initially these will entail the demonstration of association of symptoms with giving a food, and recovery when it is withdrawn, double-blind, either in repeated provocation tests on an individual, or better, by double-blind controlled trial.

87

However, not all symptoms, induced in a minority by eating a food, are food-allergic diseases (Figure 1). Food intolerance for which there is evidence of an allergic (immunological) mechanism is food-allergic disease, and that for which there is an established non-immunological mechanism (e.g. an enzyme defect) is food idiosyncrasy; if the mechanism is uncertain, the general term 'food intolerance' should be used. Each may involve the gastrointestinal tract alone or may involve many target organ systems (systemic).

Food intolerance may be to proteins, carbohydrates, fats, vitamins, and possibly other foods. The handling of patients with food idiosyncrasy may be very similar to that of food allergy, when the substance to which the patient is intolerant is an unusual molecule confined to a particular food, such as lactose. When it is an amino acid, such as phenylalanine, which is present in all proteins, the management usually differs for each one of a number of very rare diseases, usually transmitted by autosomal recessive inheritance. In this case it is therefore impossible to generalize about management, and to particularize about each disease is outside the scope of this chapter. Indeed, though the mechanisms of these diseases are splendidly reviewed by Stanbury *et al.* (1978), we are not aware of a satisfactory general review of the complexities of their management, which are the bases of several subspecialist disciplines.

Because of our uncertainty about diagnosis, it is impossible to be sure of the prevalence of food-allergic disease. But infantile eczema, which is probably largely food allergy (Atherton *et al.*, 1978), affects 3 per cent of infants and infantile colic, which some suggest is food allergy (Jakobsson and Linberg, 1978) is even commoner. There are many other symptoms established as due to food allergy (Gerrard, 1980), so the prevalence is very high in infancy and childhood, clearly higher than in adult life. This is consistent with the natural history of most childhood food allergy, which has a tendency to recover or improve, and strongly suggests that food antigens are particularly liable to induce a damaging sensitization in infancy.

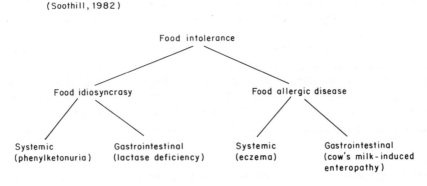

FIGURE 1   Food-allergic disease and food idiosyncrasy.

HANDLING OF FOOD ANTIGENS

There is good evidence that food antigens enter the circulation, and that they provoke immune responses, so the problem for immunologists is not why some individuals develop food allergy, but why we do not all die of it. In neonates of some species, the gastrointestinal tract readily permits access of maternal IgG passively transferred in the milk; this permeability usually ceases (gut closure) in a week or two under the influence of milk hormones In humans, the passive transfer of IgG is across the placenta, and gut permeability is mature at full-term birth; there is evidence, however, that a form of gut closure occurs at about 30 weeks gestation (Robertson et al., 1982).

The immunological aspects of infant feeding are complex (Soothill, 1982). The immune system, though largely competent after the early weeks of foetal life, is normally not active until after birth, largely because of the lack of antigen stimulus. Following contact with antigen, including ingestion, a response occurs and the immunoglobulins rise. When a food is first eaten, it is detectable in the blood, and then antibody to it appears (Lippard et al., 1936). That antibody is largely IgA. However, this response is subject to elaborate control mechanisms. Only a very small amount of food antigen enters the bloodstream in adults who have previously eaten the food; much of it is incorporated into IgA-containing complexes (Paganelli et al., 1981). Those who have not eaten the food previously have yet to acquire this protective response (immune exclusion) and absorb much more (Walker et al., 1972). Ingestion of antigen also induces partial immunological tolerance to subsequent parenteral contact with the antigen (Chase, 1946). These three responses, which occur at the same time to the same antigen, are under genetic control and can vary — apparently to some extent independently — even to the same antigen. It also appears that tolerance, and possibly immune exclusion, can be influenced by such environmental factors as nutrition (Swarbrick et al., 1978).

Mother's milk itself is probably not antigenic to the infant, but it may convey antigens to the infant from the food the mother has eaten (Kaplan and Solli, 1979). This may certainly trigger allergic symptoms such as eczema in the already sensitized infant and may possibly itself cause sensitization.

CRITERIA

Because of the insecurity of diagnosis of food intolerance in children, Goldman et al. (1963) recommended that, for research purposes, the diagnosis of milk allergy should be confined to those with symptoms which are present while the child is taking the food and disappear when the child stops taking the food, and that these observations should be confirmed three times; in addition, relevant idiosyncrasies (e.g. lactose intolerance) must be excluded. This regimen is not indicated for clinical purposes, but it usefully indicates one aspect of the complexities of the diagnosis. Conversely, however, since this takes a long time, and infants with food allergy recover, some will recover before the final cycle and so will be classed as negative; food allergy is likely to be more common than such regimens will diagnose. Some symptoms which have satisfied these criteria are listed in Table 1.

TABLE 1   Symptoms of food allergy

Systemic	Anaphylaxis, sudden death
Gastrointestinal	Vomiting, diarrhoea
Secondary to intestinal disease	Anaemia, oedema, failure to thrive
Skin	Urticaria, angioedema, eczema
Respiratory	Rhinitis, asthma
CNS	Migraine, behaviour disorder
Possible food allergy	Arthritis, enuresis, etc.

Despite such evidence of food allergy, scepticism exists, and, for educational reasons double-blind controlled trials in which effects of diet are clearly established in groups of patients are needed. The first, in eczema (Atherton *et al.*, 1978) adopted a simple empirical approach of double-blind placebo administration or withdrawal of two foods thought to be specially important — eggs and cow's milk — and showed a highly significant effect; on this regimen about one-third recover, and another third improve.

More sophisticated trials are now in hand for patients with eczema not responding adequately to diets avoiding eggs, cow's milk, chicken, beef, and individually suspected antigens, and with migraine and other possible food allergies. In these, an oligoantigenic diet (see below — a diet containing few antigens) is instituted, and, if the patient improves, foods are readministered one by one, until relapse occurs. The food is then withdrawn and it and a placebo are then readministered in a random order, with double-blind assessment of symptoms (Soothill, 1982). Much more such trial information will be needed before the scope of the subject is clearly established. Management of individual patients will always be particularized, but it will often be based on this regimen.

Following the demonstration that foods induce the symptoms, the distinction between allergy and idiosyncrasy is usually indirect. Where the symptoms are provoked by many antigenically distinct foods which contain the same non-antigenic constituent, as in phenylketonuria, an idiosyncrasy is probable. In patients with other allergic diseases, or with tests suggesting that the patient is allergic, allergy is most likely. However, since cow's milk allergy and disaccharide intolerance may exist together in a post-gastroenteritis immunodeficient, allergic child (Harrison *et al.*, 1976), the distinction may not be easy and it is not clear for many forms of food intolerance.

TYPES AND MECHANISMS OF
FOOD ALLERGIC DISEASE

Most food-allergic diseases (Table 1) occur in atopic subjects, the one-third of the population with the genetically determined, antigen-non-specific propensity for a damaging response to certain antigens—mainly inhalant and food (see below for mechanisms). This propensity is recognized by the immediate skin-prick test, which is largely an IgE-mediated process, but atopics have increased levels of IgG and IgA antibody (Platts-Mills, 1979) and probably abnormalities of other systems, so the pathogenesis of food allergy and other symptoms in atopics is not necessarily by IgE. The food-allergic diseases which atopics experience include urticaria (which may result from ingested food, or food contact on the skin), angioedema, vomiting, and anaphylactic collapse, all of which may well be IgE-mediated. Rhinitis and asthma, which may entail either direct contact with the food in the respiratory tract, or possibly systemic dissemination, may sometimes be IgE-mediated, but there is no evidence that eczema is.

Coeliac disease, though not associated with atopy, is also genetically determined, though less precisely, in that it is familial, and linked to tissue type A1, B8 and DRW3. The mechanism of damage is uncertain, but there is evidence that T cells can mediate damage similar to the villous atrophy which is seen (Ferguson and Parrott, 1973). There is indirect evidence for antibody- and complement-mediated damage in some patients with the rather slower intestinal symptoms seen in some atopics—activation and consumption of C3 (Matthew and Soothill, 1970) and deposition of immunoglobulin-, antigen-, and complement-containing complexes in the submucosal tissue (Shiner *et al.*, 1975). This mechanism would be an attractive explanation for the red cell and protein loss, presumably colonic, which may result from food allergy (Wilson *et al.*, 1974; Waldmann *et al.*, 1967). The association of colitis with food allergy has been a debated topic since Acheson and Truelove (1961) noted its association with artificial infant-feeding, but the assumption that this indicated food allergy as a cause of adult ulcerative colitis is insecure. However, most ulcerative colitis below the age of a year is food allergy (Jenkins *et al.*, 1982) and some in older children is, so the possibility should always be considered. As with most food allergy, the mechanism of damage is uncertain, but the antibody and complement-mediated ones present an attractive possibility.

FOODS PROVOKING ALLERGY

Almost any food protein can elicit allergy, and carbohydrates, lipids, and other simple molecules may elicit intolerance, sometimes known to be an idiosyncrasy (e.g. galactose), but sometimes of uncertain mechanism (intolerance)—e.g. the commonly used yellow food colouring agent, tartrazine. Some foods commonly causing food allergy in children are listed in Table 2. Many, such as cow's milk are complex mixtures of proteins, and different milk allergic patients may react to different proteins (β-lactoglobulin is the commonest). Denaturation may influence the antigenicity of the protein (Anderson *et al.*, 1979). Eggs are apparently very sensitizing and the white more than the yolk. This probably underlies a long-standing practice of delaying introduction of egg in infant feeds, particularly the whites. Normal infant feeding and the complexities and dangers of diets are outlined by Francis (1982).

TABLE 2   Some foods commonly provoking allergy
in children

Cow's milk
Hen's eggs
Fish
Meats (beef, chicken, etc.)
Cereals (wheat, oats, rice, etc.)
Nuts
Legumes (peas, beans, soya, peanuts, etc.)
Pipped fruits (strawberries, raspberries, etc.)
Other fruit (oranges, lemons, plums, apples, etc.)
Brassicas (cabbage, cauliflower, etc.)
Tomato and potato
Onion
Chocolate
Shellfish
Colours and preservatives (tartrazine, benzoate, etc.)

PREDISPOSING FACTORS

Genetic

The familial fendency in many food allergies suggests a genetic component. The first one clearly established was the association of coeliac disease with the tissue type, HLA A1, B8, DRW3 (Solheim *et al.*, 1976). The occasional but significant association of atopy with sustained immunoglobulin deficiency, especially IgA (Kaufman and Hobbs, 1970), led to the search for a wider range of immunodeficiencies. Atopy is commonly associated with transient IgA deficiency (Taylor *et al.*, 1973) and relative defects of complement-C2, and of yeast opsonization, a function of the alternative pathway of complement (Turner *et al.*, 1978). Defective T suppressor function (whether antigen or Ig class specific or not) may play a part and there may be T cell abnormalities in the cord blood of atopic subjects (Juto and Strannegard, 1979). Rarely such allergic symptoms as eczema may be associated with defects of neutrophil function (Hill and Quie, 1974). The interpretation of these complex associations is not yet clear, but hypotheses include defective exclusion or elimination of antigen, defective suppressor functions, defective induction of partial tolerance to ingested antigens, or defective responses to infections which play a critical adjuvant role in damaging sensitization. The association with many defects suggests that the mechanisms will not be simple. Tissue types influence the effect of such susceptibility, however, since atopics presenting with eczema (usually a food allergy) have an excess of HLA A1 and B8, unlike atopic patients who present with hay fever, who have an excess of A3 and B7 (Soothill *et al.*, 1976).

However, genetic factors are not the whole story, since the concordance of atopic allergic disease in monozygotic twins is not 100 per cent (Konig and Godfrey, 1974). The preponderance of food allergy in infancy and childhood, and the influence of time and place of birth (Soothill *et al.*, 1976) and other neonatal environmental factors (Salk *et al.*, 1974) point to the importance of adverse antigen contact in the neonatal period. It is likely that they operate at various levels between abnormal sensitization and development of the disease. Since eczema was becoming more common when artificial feeding was becoming more frequent and undertaken earlier, in the 1930s (Grulee and Sandford, 1936), it was likely that this played a part; and several recent prospective studies have shown that, in the offspring of atopic parents who are exclusively breast-fed for at least 4 months, the development of eczema is less than in those who are bottle- or mixed-fed (Matthew *et al.*, 1977). Two contradictory retrospective studies have appeared, but these are misleading; they did not take into account the potentially damaging effect of early supplementary feeds. The degree to which other food allergies are affected has not been reported, but there is some evidence of an effect on other allergies. Infantile colic, suspected by some to be a food allergy, is not affected (Hide and Guyer, 1981). The effect of breast feeding on eczema seems to persist, but the effect on IgE antibody is only transient. The mechanism is uncertain, but there is some reason to doubt whether it is simply the antigenicity of the artificial feeds, since cow's milk is only one of many inducing infantile eczema. There is evidence from cross-fostering rat experiments—where rat pups are fed on sensitized mothers—of antigen-specific suppression of IgE responses (Jarrett and Hall, 1979); this is probably an IgG effect and so is probably irrelevant for humans, since the IgG transfer is transplacental in them. However, there is also evidence of an antigen-non-specific increase of

IgE response in rat pups who receive cow's milk-based supplements as well as normal sucklings, directly comparable with what has been observed and postulated in man (Roberts and Soothill, 1982). One explanation could be a possible adjuvant effect of the abnormal Gram-negative flora in babies receiving supplementary feeds (Bullen *et al.*, 1977). Support for the importance of micro-organisms in provoking a damaging degree of sensitization comes from the observation that cow's milk protein gastrointestinal allergy can develop after gastroenteritis (bacterial or viral) in relatively IgA-deficient infants (Harrison *et al.*, 1976). Breast-feeding would probably have prevented this, either by preventing the infection or by avoiding the sensitizing antigen, or by its suppressive effect on allergic sensitization, or by all three. The antigenicity of the feed is important, since less allergy follows the use of less antigenic feeds (Manuel and Walker-Smith, 1981). The only randomized and controlled study, aimed at preventing allergy by diet, was carried out by Glaser and Johnstone (1953), and showed that less allergy (food and inhalant) developed in offspring of atopic parents who were fed with a soya-based feed than in those fed with a cow's milk-based feed. This has recently been confirmed (Moore *et al.*, 1982). However, the mechanism is still uncertain. Glaser and Johnston also advised mothers to avoid dairy products, which they regarded as highly sensitizing, during pregnancy. Such a measure assumes antenatal sensitization, for which there is little evidence at present, but more work on this is needed. We (Johnstone and Soothill, 1980) regard breast-feeding as the first choice since it is a more physiological approach than soya. The possible indications for and dangers of special maternal diets during lactation need more study. The role of infant feeding in non-atopic food allergy has been less studied, but it is possible that damaging sensitization may occur in the genetically vulnerable, and so may predispose to many other diseases. There is an exciting impression that coeliac disease has occurred less in Britain since breast-feeding became more common again, and since the early (before 4 months) introduction of solid feeds was abandoned (Littlewood *et al.*, 1980), suggesting that this may be such an effect. The association of ulcerative colitis with artificial feeding (Acheson and Truelove, 1961; Whorwell *et al.*, 1979) suggests that this may possibly be another example, even if it is only the infantile form of ulcerative colitis which is likely to be a food allergy.

DIAGNOSIS

The diagnosis is suspected when appropriate symptoms (Table 1) occur, but many of these have many causes (e.g. diarrhoea, or failure to thrive). All infants with some of the other symptoms, such as infantile eczema, should be assumed to have food allergy in planning initial management. The only conclusive test is the effect (see below) of an appropriate avoidance diet, preferably with at least one double-blind placebo provocation test of re-introduction of the food, provided that the symptoms are not life-threatening (anaphylaxis or angioedema leading to respiratory obstruction). For the provocation test the food is given in standard serving amounts, mixed with other foods to which the child is not allergic (Soothill, 1982) or in capsules (this is possible only for older children, and for components of foods taken in small quantities, such as colouring agents). Alternatively, an indistinguishable control preparation is given. Since severe reactions will occur rapidly, the patients should be watched for 30 minutes.

The suspicion that a disease is food allergy will be strengthened if the child also has other clearly allergic symptoms (eczema, asthma, etc.), a history of food allergy in first-degree relatives, or if the child is atopic (i.e. reacts with weal and flare to one or more of the following prick tests: *Dermatophagoides pteronyssinus*, a grass pollen, cat dander, cladosporium, cow's milk and eggs). Detection of relative immunoglobulin deficiency, the yeast opsonizing defect, eosinophilia, or a raised serum IgE will strengthen the suspicion. Since some food allergy is relieved by oral disodium cromoglycate, it may be used diagnostically too (Wraith *et al.*, 1979); improvement of symptoms following its use supports the case for food allergy, and justifies a further search for the offending food. These tests suggest that the symptoms are in the general category of food allergy, although tests to find which allergens cause symptoms in such a subject are less satisfactory; knowledge of likely ones (Table 2) and a careful history of the association of symptoms and diet, are the most effective. An indication may come from a dislike of a food (which may still be taken in cooked foods) or a particular craving, or if the child describes an odd sensation in his mouth when he takes the food. Often, however, one must take recourse to the empirical approach of the oligoantigenic diet (see below). Some extra information is obtained from skin-prick tests with suspected foods, but these may be positive to foods which do not induce symptoms in the patient, and skin tests may be negative to some which do. There have been many claims for tests for antibody (agglutinating, precipitating, etc.) but there is no clear evidence of the usefulness of these, and the only claim that IgE antibody may be positive when the skin test is negative is that of Munro *et al.* (1980) in migraine. Lymphocyte responses are probably too cumbersome and their usefulness is not established.

In coeliac disease, diagnosis has depended on the demonstration of total or sub-total villous atrophy by intestinal biopsy, with recovery on withdrawal of gluten from the diet. The demonstration of similar, if less severe damage in cow's milk allergy (Kuitenen *et al.*, 1973), and in fish, rice, and chicken allergy (Vitoria *et al.*, 1982) stresses that this is not an antigen-specific phenomenon, and since some patients with food-allergic diarrhoea have normal intestinal biopsies, the habit of intestinal biopsy in all such cases seems irrational. Recovery of symptoms will be the main criterion of success for antigen avoidance treatment, but for intestinal allergy, a search for faecal eosinophils and Charcot–Leyden crystals may have a role, and so many colonoscopy.

MANAGEMENT

In inhalant allergy in children, allergen-specific treatment (avoidance or hyposensitization) have little potential and only a limited role; symptomatic relief by drugs is the first line. In food allergy antigen avoidance is easier, and is the mainstay of treatment, but diets are difficult, socially disruptive, and potentially dangerous. Local drug treatment is effective in eczema, and may be all that is needed in mild cases, though systemic steroids and excessive use of strong local steroids should be avoided. However, severe acute reactions may occur to foods, as to other allergens, which may require urgent effective use of drugs.

Emergency treatment of anaphylaxis and respiratory obstruction

Anaphylaxis is syncopal collapse following contact with antigen, usually by ingestion or injection; this may also induce respiratory obstruction due to angioedema of the pharynx and larynx. The prime treatment of these highly dangerous medical emergencies is adrenaline — the intramuscular injection of adrenaline 1 in 1000 0.5 ml, repeated if necessary after 10 minutes. The dose need not be modified for weight. Consideration should be given in severe cases of intravenous adrenaline 1 in 10,000 0.1 ml/kg. Intravenous resuscitation, intravenous hydrocortisone (100 mg) and intravenous chlorpheniramine (Piriton, 0.2 mg/kg) may be used as secondary measures. The respiratory obstruction of angioedema may require oxygen and intubation. Tracheostomy is rarely needed.

Prevention

The standard regimen, applicable to all healthy infants, but specially recommended for offspring of atopic parents, is exclusive breast-feeding (thirst quenched with additional water or dextrose solution if required) for 4 months. Following this, particularly in families with marked cow's milk allergy, weaning may avoid milk products until 1 year. It is desirable to maintain partial breast-feeding for some further months, but if this is stopped, a soya-based preparation (e.g. Cow and Gate Formula S, or prosobee) may be used. Eggs may also be avoided. Vitamin supplements can be introduced at this stage. This regimen does not differ significantly from that recommended for normal infants (DHSS, 1980). However, premature, jaundiced and hypoglycaemic babies require special management.

  Should breast-feeding be impracticable, soya preparations (see above) should be used. Goat's milk is not a satisfactory human milk substitute below the age of 1 year.

Vulnerable infants recovering from gastroenteritis may initially be fed with preparations which are less sensitizing, such as pregestimil. Secondary disaccharide intolerance is also important.

Antigen avoidance diets

Many infants and children who are allergic to foods are effectively treated by avoidance of a single or a few foods (e.g. cow's milk avoidance in infantile gastrointestinal cow's milk allergy, or avoidance of milk, eggs, chicken, beef, and known antigens to which the child is sensitive in eczema (Soothill, 1982). Appropriate milk substitutes are the soya feeds or pregestimil, mentioned above, or goat's milk for older children; but some may react to any one of these. Beside avoidance of particular foods, the avoidance of certain categories of foods may sometimes be useful. Intolerance may occur (the evidence for allergy is not clear) to a range of additives in factory-produced foods, especially colours (e.g. tartrazine) and preservatives (e.g. benzoates), and the simplest way of diagnosing and treating such disorders is a diet avoiding all factory-produced food, with a double-blind provocation when the child is improved, to confirm the diagnosis. However, this too is difficult; people forget that butter and cheese often contain colours. The principles of diets in infants and children are outlined by Francis (1982). Some, especially older children with slower reactions to many foods (e.g. eczema or migraine), will require a more complex dietary approach. Giving an oligoantigenic diet for 2 weeks (Soothill, 1982) containing only a few antigenically different foods (e.g. based on lamb, potatoes, beans and peas, soya 'milk', apple, sugar, colour-free vitamins, minerals, and water) may be associated with a dramatic improvement. Foods are then reintroduced one by one, at weekly intervals; when symptoms recur that food is withdrawn, and may be reintroduced, double-blind with a placebo, either as an individual confirmatory provocation, or as part of a double-blind controlled trial. It should be stressed that such diets are very difficult, particularly when factory-processed foods are used; only a sophisticated mother recognizes that calcium caseinate is milk.

Since children usually outgrow their food allergy, avoided foods should be reintroduced periodically—say 1 year after the last symptom, starting with small quantities, under appropriate supervision.

All such treatments are potentially dangerous and should be supervised by experienced paediatricians and dietitians. Many infants are now being placed on dangerously inadequate diets (Tripp et al., 1979). Also, the reintroduction of a food, accidental or intentional, may be associated with anaphylaxis or respiratory obstruction. Fortunately, individual patients tend to continue to react with the same symptoms as they had before. Children with eczema will relapse with eczema, and children with angioedema will relapse with angioedema, but there are exceptions. The first dose of a reintroduced food should often be given under observation, and the things required for treatment of anaphylaxis, etc., should be available (see above). Diets are also socially disruptive, and should be undertaken only when the symptom is bad enough to warrant it, and when a clear-cut diagnosis has been made, usually involving at least one double-blind placebo challenge.

There is much loose assertion of vague symptoms being associated to allergy to a very widespread range of foods and other substances. It is likely that some of the patients for whom benefit is claimed for diets are hysterical. These aspects should be approach with caution but they should not distract from the common need of antigen-avoidance diets in the wide range of common, readily confirmable food allergic diseases.

Drugs

Apart from the use of drugs in emergencies (see above), drugs play a smaller part than for inhalant allergy, but oral disodium cromoglycate (dissolve and hold in the mouth for some minutes before swallowing) is of benefit (Wraith *et al.*, 1979), particularly in patients who have benefited partly from diet. In infants and children, the strict diet is the main line of management, and this and the other interesting drugs which influence the local allergic response in the gut such as aspirin and indomethacin (Lessof *et al.*, 1979) have been less appraised in children, and probably have only a minor role. Local skin or inhalation treatment appropriate for eczema and asthma are outlined in appropriate dermatological and respiratory texts.

REFERENCES

Acheson, E. D., and Truelove, S. C. (1961). Early weaning in the aetiology of ulcerative colitis. *Br. Med. J.*, **2**, 929.

Anderson, K. J., McLaughlin, P., Devey, M. E., and Coombs, R. R. A. (1979). Anaphylactic sensitivity of guinea pigs drinking different preparations of cows milk and infant formulae. *Clin. Exp. Immunol.*, **35**, 454.

Atherton, D. J., Sewell, M., Soothill, J. F., Wells, R. S., and Chilvers, C. E. D. (1978). A double blind cross-over trial of an antigen avoidance diet in atopic eczema. *Lancet*, **1**, 402.

Bullen, C. L., Tearle, P. V., and Steward, M. G. (1977). The effect of 'humanized' milks and supplemented breast feeding on the faecal flora of infants. *J. Med. Microbiol.*, **10**, 404.

Chase, M. W. (1946). Inhibition of experimental drug allergy by prior feeding of the sensitizing agent. *Proc. Soc. Exp. Biol. Med.*, **61**, 257.

DHSS (Department of Health and Social Security) (1980). Present day practice in infant feeding. *Rep. Health Soc. Lab.*, **18**. HMSO, London.

Ferguson, A., and Parrott, D. M. V. (1973). Histopathology and time course of rejection of allografts of mouse small intestine. *Transplantation*, **15**, 546.

Francis, D. E. M. (1982). *Diets for Sick Children*. 4th edition. (In preparation.) Blackwell Scientific Publications, Oxford.

Gerrard, J. W. (1980). In: *Food Allergy—New Prospectives* (ed. Gerrard, J. W.). Charles C. Thomas, Springfield, Illinois.

Glaser, J., and Johnstone, D. E. (1953). Prophylaxis of allergic disease in newborns. *J. Am. Med. Assoc.*, **153**, 620.

Goldman, A. S., Anderson, D. W., Sellars, W. A., Saperstein, S., Kniker, W. T., Halpern, S. R. *et al.* (1963). Milk allergy. (1) Oral challenge with milk and isolated milk proteins in allergic children. *Pediatrics*, **32**, 425.

Grulee, C., and Sandford, H. (1936). The influence of breast feeding and artificial feeding in infantile eczema. *J. Pediatr.*, **9**, 223.

Harrison, M., Kilby, A., Walker-Smith, J. A., France, N. E., and Wood, C. B. S. (1976). Cows milk protein intolerance; possible association with gastroenteritis, lactose intolerance and IgA deficiency. *Br. Med. J.*, **1**, 1501.

Hide, D. W., and Guyer, B. M. (1981). Clinical manifestations of allergy related to breast and cows milk feeding in an infant population. *Arch. Dis. Childh.*, **56**, 172.

Hill, H. R., and Quie, P. (1974). Raised serum IgE levels and defective neutrophil chemotaxis in three children with eczema and recurrent bacterial infection. *Lancet*, **1**, 183.

Jakobsson, I., and Linberg, T. (1978). Cows milk as a cause of infantile colic in breast fed infants. *Lancet*, **2**, 437.

Jarrett, E. E., and Hall, E. (1979). Selective suppression of IgE antibody responsiveness by maternal influence. *Nature*, **280**, 145.

Jenkins, H. R., Harries, J. T., Pincott, J., and Soothill, J. F. (1982). (In preparation.)

Johnstone, D. E., and Soothill, J. F. (1980). Prevention of allergic disease. In: *Allergic Diseases of Infancy, Childhood and Adolescence*. (eds C. W. Bierman and D. S. Pearlman). Saunders, Philadelphia, p.346.

Juto, R., and Strannegard, O. (1979). T lymphocytes and blood eosinophils in early infancy in relation to heredity for allergy and type of feeding. *J. Allergy Clin. Immunol.*, **64**, 38.

Kaplan, M. S., and Solli, N. J. (1979). Immunoglobulin E in breast fed atopic children. *J. Allergy Clin. Immunol.*, **64**, 22.

Kaufman, H., and Hobbs, J. R. (1970). Immunoglobulin deficiencies in an atopic population. *Lancet*, **2**, 1061.

Konig, P., and Godfrey, S. (1974). Exercise-induced bronchial lability in monozygotic (identical) and dizygotic (non-identical) twins. *J. Allergy. Clin. Immunol.*, **54**, 280.

Kuitunen, P., Rapola, J., Savilahti, E., and Visikorpi, J. K. V. (1973). Response of the jejunal mucosa to cows milk in the malabsorption syndrome with cows milk intolerance. *Acta Paediat. Scand.*, **62**, 585.

Lessof, M. H., Buisseret, P. D., Merrett, J., Wraith, D. G., and Youlten, L. J. F. (1979). Mechanisms involving prostaglandins in food intolerance. In: *The Mast Cell; its role in health and disease* (eds J. Pepys and A. M. Edwards). Pitman Medical, Tunbridge Wells, p.406.

Lippard, V. M., Schloss, O. M., and Johnson, P. A. (1936). Immune reactions induced in infants by intestinal absorption of incompletely digested cows milk protein. *Am. J. Dis. Child.*, **51**, 562.

Littlewood, J. M., Crollick, A. J., and Richards, I. D. G. (1980). Childhood coeliac disease is disappearing. *Lancet*, **2**, 1359.

Manuel, P. D., and Walker-Smith, J. (1981). A comparison of three infant feeding formulae for the prevention of delayed recovery after infantile gastroenteritis. *Acta Paediatr. Belg.*, **34**, 13.

Matthew, D. J., Taylor, B., Norman, A. P., Turner, M. W., and Soothill, J. F. (1977). Prevention of eczema. *Lancet*, **1**, 321.

Matthews, T. S., and Soothill, J. F. (1970). Complement activation after milk feeding in children with cows milk allergy. *Lancet*, **2**, 893.

Moore, W. J., Colley, J. R. T., Midwinter, R. E., Turner, M. W., and Soothill, J. F. (1982). (In preparation.)

Munro, J., Brostoff, J., Carini, C., and Zilkha, K. (1980). Food allergy in migraine. *Lancet*, **2**, 1.

Paganelli, R., Levinsky, R. J., and Atherton, D. J. (1981). Detection of specific antigen within immune complexes. Validation of the assay and its application to food antigen antibody complexes in healthy and food allergic subjects. *Clin. Exp. Immunol.*, **46**, 44.

Platts-Mills, T. A. E. (1979). Local production of IgG, IgA and IgE antibodies in grass pollen hay fever. *J. Immunol.*, **122**, 2218.

Robertson, D., Paganelli, R., Dinwiddie, R., and Levinsky, R. J. (1982). Milk antigen absorption in the premature and term neonate. *Arch. Dis. Childh.*, **57**, 369.

Roberts, S. A., and Soothill, J. F. (1982). Provocation of allergic response by supplementary feeds of cows milk. *Arch. Dis. Childh.*, **57**, 127.

Salk, L., Grellong, B. A., Straus, W., and Dietrich, J. (1974). Perinatal complications in the history of asthmatic children. *Am. J. Dis. Child.*, **127**, 30.

Shiner, M., Ballard, J., and Smith, M. E. (1975). The small intestinal mucosa in cow's milk allergy. *Lancet*, **1**, 136.

Solheim, B. G., Ek, J., Thune, P. O., Baklien, K., Bratlie, A., Rankin, B., Thoresen, A. B., and Thorsby, E. (1976). HLA antigens in dermatitis herpetiformis and coeliac disease. *Tissue Antigens*, **7**, 57.

Soothill, J. F. (1982). The atopic child. In: *Paediatric Clinical Immunology* (eds J. F. Soothill, A. R. Hayward, and C. B. S. Wood). Blackwell, Oxford. (In press.)

Soothill, J. F., Stokes, C. R., Turner, M. W., Norman, A. P., and Taylor, B. (1976). Predisposing factors and the development of reaginic allergy in infancy. *Clin. Allergy*, **6**, 305.

Stanbury, J. B., Wyngaarden, J. B., and Fredrickson, D. S. (1978). *The Metabolic Basis of Inherited Disease*, 4th edn. McGraw-Hill, New York.

Swarbrick, E. T., Stokes, C. R., and Soothill, J. F. (1978). The absorption of antigens after oral immunization and the simultaneous induction of specific systemic tolerance. *Gut*, **20**, 121.

Taylor, B., Norman, A. P., Orgel, H. A., Stokes, C. R., Turner, M. W., and Soothill, J. F. (1973). Transient IgA deficiency and pathogenesis of infantile atopy. *Lancet*, **2**, 111.

Tripp, J. H., Francis, D. E. M., Knight, J. A., and Harries, J. T. (1979). Infant feeding practices; a cause for concern. *Br. Med. J.*, **2**, 707.

Turner, M. W., Mowbray, J. F., Harvey, B. A. M., Brostoff, J., Wells, R. S., and Soothill, J. F. (1978). Defective yeast opsonization and C2 deficiency in atopic patients. *Clin. Exp. Immunol.*, **34**, 253

Vitoria, J. C., Camarero, C., Sojo, A., Ruiz, A., and Rodriguez-Soriano, J. (1982). Enteropathy related to fish, rice and chicken. *Arch. Dis. Childh.*, **57**, 44.

Waldmann, T. A., Wochner, R. D., Laster, L., and Gordon, R. S. (1967). Allergic gastroenteropathy. A cause of excessive gastrointestinal protein loss. *N. Engl. J. Med.*, **276**, 762.

Walker, W. A., Isselbacher, K. J., and Bloch, K. J. (1972). Intestinal uptake of macromolecules; effect of oral immunization. *Science*, **177**, 608.
Whorwell, P. J., Holdstock, G., Whorwell, G. M., and Wright, R. (1979). Bottle feeding, early gastroenteritis and inflammatory bowel disease. *Br. Med. J.*, **1**, 382.
Wilson, J. F., Lahey, M. E., and Heiner, D. C. (1974). Studies in iron metabolism. V. Further observations on cows milk-induced gastrointestinal bleeding in infants with iron deficiency anaemia. *J. Pediatr.*, **84**, 335.
Wraith, D. G., Young, G. V. W., and Lee, T. H. (1979). The management of food allergy with diet and Nalcrom. In: *The Mast Cell; its role in health and disease* (eds J. Pepys and A. M. Edwards). Pitman Medical, Tunbridge Wells, p.443.

Reactions to Food in Adults

M. H. Lessof

Professor of Medicine
Guy's Hospital Medical School, London

In the adult, as in the child, a wide range of symptoms has been attributed to food reactions, and a number of extravagant claims have been made. When faced with the more bizarre effects which have been described, the most common view among the medical profession has been one of scepticism or of total disbelief. The problem has been exacerbated by the lack of a clear definition of the difference between food fads, immunologically determined food-allergic diseases, and food intolerance which can be due to a pharmacological or toxic action. In addition there may be an idiosyncrasy of the host, either based on enzyme defects or of unknown cause.

One of the problems has been the paucity of reliable diagnostic tests, and this has sometimes led to an uncritical use of the term 'food allergy' by authors when referring to even the most vaguely defined intolerance to specific foods. Patients with psychiatric or gastrointestinal diseases of almost any type may notice that unpleasant symptoms can follow the ingestion of particular foods in quite modest quantities. Such a history by itself is clearly of limited value. The terms in current use (see Chapter 2) therefore need to be clarified.

In reaching a diagnosis of food-allergic disease two criteria need to be satisfied. The first is that a true food intolerance can be demonstrated—as shown by a recurrence of symptoms on two or more occasions when a specific food is taken. The second is the presence of an immunological component to the patient's disease.

Perhaps the most difficult task is to establish the presence of a true food intolerance in cases where the symptoms are subjective only, especially if those symptoms suggest psychiatric ill-health. Since it is clear that psychological complications may arise when the administered food is identifiable by the patient, a blind challenge through a nasogastric tube is necessary wherever there is any possibility of doubt. To establish the presence of an immunological

103

aspect of the illness is hardly less difficult, but may be suggested by the presence of such allergic manifestations as urticaria or asthma. Further evidence can be provided by means of skin tests or laboratory evidence for the presence of specific antibodies to foods. Finally, there may be a need to demonstrate that the results of a challenge with the appropriate food involve a significant immunological reaction, or that the response can be modified specifically by anti-allergic measures.

Food intolerance

Where there is no evidence of an immunological process, the precise nature of food intolerance remains uncertain, even when its presence is confirmed by repeated challenge. Symptoms such as vomiting, diarrhoea, headache, joint pains, and general malaise are by no means confined to allergic subjects. Tachycardia which develops after the compulsive drinking of tea or coffee (Finn and Cohen, 1978) suggests a direct pharmacological effect of caffeine. Abdominal pain after drinking milk can have more than one cause and may be due to lactose intolerance, which is common in some communities (Blumenthal et al., 1981). The headache which can follow the drinking of small amounts of wine may be provoked by histamine (Kalish, 1981) or by other agents which are released when the wine is allowed to stand after it has been opened (Kaufman, 1981). Moneret-Vautrin (1979) has suggested that histamine-rich foods, such as fermented cheeses, canned foods, and sausages, can also induce reactions which can mimic allergy to the point of inducing skin reactions of urticarial type. The same is true of certain histamine-releasing or tyramine-containing foods, such as chocolate, cheese and canned fish.

The relstionship between specific food intolerance and migraine or other types of headache has been reviewed in Chapter 8.

Allergy or toxicity

In general, where a reaction is caused by very small quantities of the offending material, it is likely that an allergic basis will be found. On the other hand, reactions to food additives such as monosodium gluta-mate (Kwok, 1968) may be simply toxic effects. It is also claimed that toxins such as polychlorinated biphenyl, colouring agents such as tartrazine, and preservatives such as benzoic acid can cause toxic reactions (Lockey, 1972).

The incidence of clinical reactions to toxins, and also to contaminated food materials, is probably much higher than is generally realized. The toxic effects of chemical agents in food come to light most dramatically when they cause outbreaks—in epidemic form—of unexplained illness or death. Mild and sporadic cases undoubtedly occur but are much more difficult to identify, especially if they also depend on the susceptibility of selected members of the population. In the recent outbreak of a 'toxic–allergic' syndrome due to contaminated rape-seed oil (Tabuenca, 1981), symptoms as varied as fever, rash, muscle pain, headache, and drowsiness were combined with evidence of interstitial pneumonitis, lymphadenopathy, hepatosplenomegaly, cerebral oedema, and eosinophilia; and 43 per cent had a raised serum IgE level. A chronic phase often followed, possibly caused by the release of toxic oleoanilides from damaged cells. Nevertheless some members of the affected families, although exposed to the contaminated oil, either escaped altogether or recovered after developing acute but transient symptoms; but females who had the tissue type HLA DR3 or DR4 were particularly prone to progress to the chronic phase of this disorder (Vicario et al., 1982). Such examples as this 'Spanish oil syndrome' serve merely to emphasize how individual susceptibility to contaminated food can vary, even in severe disorders where the cause is known. When the symptoms are mild and more insidious, the difficulties of detection and of diagnosis are considerably greater.

The complex relationship between reactions to chemical substances and to drugs adds a further complication. Patients who respond to artificial colours often also have an aspirin idiosyncrasy. It has not, however, been conclusively shown whether such reactions are a pharmacological idiosyncrasy or due either to a toxic or an immunological cause (Stenius and Lemola, 1976; Harnett et al., 1978).

In the case of aspirin, there is by no means always a high serum IgE level or other conclusive evidence of an allergic response. On clinical grounds alone, however, aspirin reactions such as asthma, rhinitis, or eczema suggest an allergic origin. In a series of 205 patients with aspirin sensitivity who were studied by Speer and his colleagues (1981), as many as 133 had urticaria or angioedema, 73 had asthma, and the series included two patients who developed anaphylactic shock. In addition, 90 per cent were sensitive to inhalants, foods, and/or other drugs, including 153 (74 per cent) who reacted to at least one food. While a relationship between aspirin idiosyncrasy and food intolerance has long been attributed to the salicylate content of some vegetable substances, the foods which caused reactions in this series included milk in 97 and chocolate in 62, in addition to citrus fruits, tomato, egg, corn, legumes, pork, shellfish, food dyes, and miscellaneous vegetable materials. The authors note that a suppression of prostaglandin synthesis or an increased synthesis of other arachidonic acid metabolites could not easily explain this close association with food reactions; nor could it explain the even higher incidence of reactions to inhaled allergens. There is still no agreement about how to distinguish an idiosyncrasy to aspirin from an immunological reaction to this drug.

Reactions to foods and to drugs may thus coexist in the same subject, with features which suggest both idiosyncrasy and allergy. Establishing the precise mechanism may be difficult. Even when a food reaction is clearly allergic in nature and accompanied by a high serum IgE level and clinical features which suggest allergy, it is not always the food itself which is responsible. Contaminating levels of drugs or antibiotics are a recognized cause of problems, for example in those patients who react to traces of penicillin in the milk of penicillin-treated cows. There may also be a reaction to contaminants such as aflatoxin resulting from a growth of aspergillus mould on grains of various kinds, or on beans or peanuts (Fries, 1981).

Cross-sensitization provides a further problem and ensures that allergic reactions, even to a single protein, can be provoked by more than one food. Soya beans, which are now widely used in plastics and in various manufactured materials, can sensitize to all of these substances but also to botanically related legumes such as peas, beans and lentils (Fries, 1971). Some foods have, nevertheless, a very strong tendency to sensitize. Most reports emphasize egg, milk, fish, and wheat as being important, and many give a prominent place to chocolate and soft fruit (Speer, 1973). Other foods have also been incriminated (see Table 1); in all, many hundreds have been reported as a cause of symptoms in occasional patients.

TABLE 1   Main foods causing symptoms of intolerance*

Milk (46)	Fish/shellfish (22)
Egg (40)	Wheat/flour (9)
Nuts/peanuts (22)	Chocolate (8)

Also: artificial colours   (7)
         pork/bacon   (7)
         chicken, tomato, soft fruits, and cheese   (6 each)

Of the 20 other foods invoked, yeast or 'Marmite' was mentioned four times; tea and coffee twice

*Based on a series of 100 patients (Lessof et al., 1980b)

The exact nature of the allergen in particular foods is still a subject for investigation. The reaction to certain fish such as cod and shrimp appear to be provoked by specific proteins which have now been characterized (Aas and Lundkvist, 1973; Hoffman et al., 1981), but the response to other foods may depend on a variety of ingredients which are not necessarily the same in every case. The diagnosis of allergy to wheat products may at one time have involved an element of confusion, until the technique of jejunal biopsy allowed a diagnosis of coeliac disease to be made in many of these cases. However, gluten-sensitive diarrhoea can certainly occur without any evidence of coeliac disease (Cooper *et al.*, 1980) and there are, in addition, patients who appear to react only to white flour or to processed wheat products.

Although it is a problem that mainly concerns children, there is much to be learnt from milk allergy, which has been studied more than any other food reaction. There are at least 20 proteins in milk, but casein, α-lactalbumin, β-lactoglobulin, and bovine serum albumin are responsible for most of the reactions that are observed. Reactions against single allergens are exceptional and two or more proteins are usually involved (Goldman and Heiner, 1977). Contamination of cow's milk can also occur with penicillin, other antibiotics, peanuts, and wheat (Bahna and Heiner, 1980). When milk proteins are themselves responsible for the adverse reaction, it is of considerable practical importance that heat denaturation can sometimes protect (Fries, 1947). The currently available 'long-life milk' can therefore provide a useful addition to the diet in some cases.

PATHOGENESIS OF FOOD ALLERGY

A variety of factors contribute to the pathogenesis of food-allergic disease. A lack of secretory IgA may predispose to infection or reduce the resistance of the mucosal barrier. Defects in the gut mucosa may allow an excessive absorption of large, allergenic molecules from the gut lumen. The way in which the body reacts to such molecules shows considerable variation from person to person. In members of an atopic family, a tendency to form IgE antibodies against food allergens may well predispose to this disease. In addition, conditioning factors, such as viral infection, can appear to provoke allergic reactions for the first time in previously healthy subjects (Frick *et al.*, 1979). The tendency to form immune complexes, either in unduly large quantities or of the type which persists in the circulation, may provoke allergic or inflammatory reactions in susceptible individuals (*Proceedings of the First Food Allergy Workshop*, 1980). Deficiencies of complement components such as C_2 (Turner *et al.*, 1978) or defects in the phagocytic ability of leucocytes (Soothill, 1976) can lead to an inefficient handling of immune complexes which may therefore persist in the circulation instead of being efficiently eliminated by the reticuloendothelial system. The addition of a cell-mediated response may also contribute and prolong any abnormal reactions which occur.

The abnormal physiology associated with food allergic reactions in the bowel wall has been discussed in Chapter 4. In clinical terms, food-allergic disease may be of more than one kind. If the predominant reaction is an immediate one, any associated immunological reaction is likely to involve IgE antibody to the food concerned, and it is possible to look for diagnostic evidence of an allergic disorder by testing for specific IgE antibodies or by looking, less directly, for evidence of the release of local mediators such as histamine or prostaglandins (Buisseret et al., 1978). Though the significance of this finding is still not clear, there may also be evidence of an associated defect of intestinal permeability (Jackson et al., 1981).

Where the main response is a late reaction, it is unlikely that this will be wholly dependent on IgE, or it may not involve IgE at all. Pseudo-allergic reactions may need to be excluded (see Chapter 7); but even in highly atopic subjects late reactions to the ingestion of food are not always associated with positive skin test reactions or may be associated only with a late skin response, 4–6 hours after challenge. This has given rise to the strong suspicion that IgE antibodies represent only an inconstant part of the immunological response and that IgG antibodies or other agents may be involved. A sub-class of IgG which is heat-stable at 56 °C can act as a 'short-term sensitizing antibody' for the skin or tissues, and this has also been invoked (Parish, 1978; Pepys et al., 1979). It therefore seems possible that, by detecting IgG subclass antibodies to specific foods, further diagnostic tests may be developed in the future. It has indeed been suggested that, in asthmatic subjects, the detection of IgG4 antibody to egg and milk can suggest a food-allergic cause (Gwynn et al., 1982).

The presence of circulating IgG antibodies to milk or other foods may be demonstrable in diseases such as ulcerative colitis, even where there is no evidence of an associated food intolerance (Wright and Truelove, 1965). IgG antibody to gluten has also been found in regional ileitis, without any evidence of gluten enteropathy (Unsworth et al., 1981). The suggestion has therefore been made that this type of antibody merely represents a 'mopping-up' reaction to the excessive amounts of protein which can be absorbed across an ulcerated mucous membrane. It does not of course follow that all IgG anti-food antibodies should be ignored. Exceptionally, in cases of egg white and fish sensitivity (Berrens et al., 1981), it has been possible to show that the presence of IgG antibodies to food is associated with activation of the complement series of enzymes and with clinical feature such as urticaria or asthma. Even if the presence of IgG antibodies to food components cannot directly explain the more insidious reactions to food antigens, it is possible that their effect might be mediated indirectly, by immune complex formation (Brostoff et al., 1979; Paganelli et al., 1979, 1981). Both early and late reactions might then be explicable either by different immunological mechanisms or by such other processes as the non-immunological 'pseudo-allergic' response of Moneret-Vautrin. It should be emphasized that the finding of IgG antibodies (Dannaeus et al., 1979) or of circulating immune complexes provides no proof that they have caused the patient's symptoms. Circulating immune complexes can also be found in individuals who lack symptoms of any kind (Paganelli et al., 1979, 1981); and their persistence in the circulation may depend, not on food allergy, but on a delayed clearance of immune complexes which is seen, for example, in diseases such as glomerulo-nephritis (Cairns *et al.*, 1981).

The search for other immunological mechanisms in food intolerance still continues. Clearly IgE reactions, even when they are demonstrable, do not explain all the syndromes which are encountered. For example, clinical hypersensitivity to cow's milk in infancy can lead to similar changes in the small bowel mucosa to those seen in gluten enteropathy, but it is interesting that the mucosal damage which follows a gluten challenge in the latter condition shows little evidence of an IgE response. It does, on the other hand, have histological features which suggest an Arthus reaction (Anand *et al.*, 1981). While the evidence of an immunological change in gluten enteropathy has been challenged (Cornell and Rolles, 1978), it seems unlikely that the disease could be due simply to the toxic effects of intermediate gluten metabolites. For one thing, similar mucosal changes have been described in soya protein intolerance, in which gluten effects have not been invoked (Ament and Rubin, 1972).

While immunological abnormalities are thus difficult to interpret, they clearly have a prominent role in many cases of food intolerance. Improved investigative methods are still needed, however, if we are to establish the precise part played by idiosyncrasy, pseudo-allergic and pharmacological effects, IgE and IgG reactions, immune complexes, and delayed hyper-sensitivity reactions.

DIAGNOSTIC METHODS

If it is postulated that foods are responsible for particular symptoms, the first stage in the diagnosis is to demonstrate that the symptoms disappear when the suspect food is eliminated from the diet. The most simple clinical approach to diagnosis therefore involves the use of some form of elimination diet, as discussed below in the section on management, and this can then be followed by challenge. Elimination diets may range, however, from the very simple to the very tedious. In each case the objective is to establish a dietary regime on which the patient remains symptom-free, after which the omitted foods are re-introduced in stages until a satisfactory maintenance diet is achieved or until symptoms recur. A recurrence of symptoms during the phase in which foods are being re-introduced is an indication to go back to a simpler diet. As with all dietary regimes, it is essential to ensure that the final diet achieved is one which is nutritionally adequate. The elimination diet may follow three steps:

(1) elimination of particular suspect foods (for example shellfish or milk);
(2) the introduction of an empirical 'basic exclusion diet' (excluding artificial colours, preservatives, and the more common food allergens such as milk and dairy products, eggs, fish, and nuts);

(3) in severe and uncontrolled cases (as in angioedema) the use of a very simple 'elemental' diet which aims at controlling symptoms completely by the eradication of virtually every known allergen, so that a baseline can be established on which to develop a more adequate dietary regime.

The use of inpatient observation in the investigation of suspected food allergy varies in different units. In patients with psychological symptoms who have themselves diagnosed 'food allergy', admission for psychiatric assessment and a series of dietary challenges via a nasogastric tube may offer the most simple way of demonstrating that the diagnosis has been properly considered and can (or cannot) be excluded. A fluid, 'elemental diet' is seldom needed, but if it is, the use of bottled, 'natural' water may help to identify those exceptionally rare cases of sensitivity to such widely used chemicals as the plasticizers which are even present in tap water. Preparations of the 'Vivonex' type can thus be justified on occasions, despite the fact that they are not, themselves, totally free of chemical contamination.

The effect of dietary challenge may be easier to evaluate when a patient has had a symptom-free interval while on an elimination diet. In those cases where the symptoms are clear-cut and associated with objective changes such as urticaria, angioedema, or asthma, a blind challenge is then unnecessary. In other cases, as in children with cow's milk allergy, or in gluten enteropathy at any age, a jejunal biopsy may be required to demonstrate the specific changes provoked by the suspect food.

When intolerance to a specific food has been demonstrated without clear clinical evidence of an immunological reaction, further diagnostic tests are needed before the diagnosis of food-allergic disease can be accepted.

Skin tests are simple, cheap, and are capable of giving diagnostic information within 10–15 minutes, provided that the materials used in the test have been sufficiently well standardized to lessen the chance of non-specific reactions (Lessof et al., 1980a). Where food extracts have been used to screen large numbers of people attending an allergy clinic, it has nevertheless been evident that 3–4 per cent of 'clinically false-positive' reactions are seen. In discussing this observation, Bock and his colleagues (1977) have suggested that minor degrees of hypersensitivity occur without any detectable clinical abnormality. The assertion seems the more plausible in view of the more recent validation — by means of laboratory radioallergosorbent methods — of a close correlation between skin test and laboratory evidence of an IgE antibody reaction in such cases. If further evidence were needed, for the general validity of the skin test method, this has been provided by Eriksson (1977) who showed a 77 per cent correlation between skin tests and the results of challenge tests in patients with allergy to commonly inhaled substances.

The choice between skin-prick tests and intradermal tests has been the subject of controversy, largely on a transatlantic basis. The fact remains, however, that if allowances are made for the different volumes of fluid which penetrate the epidermis (perhaps 0.05 ml for the intradermal and 10^{-6} ml for the skin-prick method—see Squire, 1952), the results are closely comparable (M. Harries, personal communication). To allow for anything from a 200- to a 1000-fold difference in the volume introduced, it is necessary to use a correspondingly more concentrated solution for skin-prick tests than for the intradermal method.

The correlation between skin methods and other tests has been much studied, but except for a few foods, including egg, nuts, fish, and sometimes milk, IgE-based tests have all fallen short of providing a reliable diagnostic method, even for patients whose clinical condition strongly suggests an immunological reaction. In such cases these tests may appear to lack both sensitivity and specificity. To some extent this may have resulted from the use of crude food extracts which either contain insufficient antigen or, on the other hand, include materials which are capable of provoking non-specific histamine release. Another problem, however, has arisen from the assumption that an IgE-mediated process should be looked for in all immunological reactions, whatever their nature and their time-scale.

Leucocyte histamine release tests have been much studied (Bock et al., 1977) but remain cumbersome and not always reliable. Radioallergosorbent tests (RASTs) and comparable laboratory tests for IgE antibodies are, on the other hand, capable of great sensitivity. While they still have problems because of the non-specific positive results which are caused, for example, by lectins or by particular vegetable foods, these are gradually being resolved. With improvements in technology and with the discovery of cross-reacting carbohydrate determinants in a variety of vegetables (Aalberse et al., 1981), rapid improvements in the results of IgE-based laboratory tests may be expected.

Antibodies of classes other than IgE are also currently under study, as are food antigen-containing immune complexes in which immunoglobulins of various classes may be found (Paganelli et al., 1981). However, skin tests and RASTs remain by far the most useful tests for the clinician.

The limitations of skin-prick tests and RASTs have been discussed elsewhere (Lessof, 1981). It is clear that improvements will be needed, both in test materials and in diagnostic methods, if these aids to diagnosis are to be used with confidence.

CLINICAL FEATURES

Such features as vomiting and anaphylactic shock can develop within minutes, and in infancy can be provoked by less than a millilitre of milk (Savilahti, 1981). A variety of other symptoms may occur (Figure 1), including abdominal symptoms such as pain, bloating, and constipation. In addition there may be a more widespread allergic reaction.

TIME COURSE OF SYMPTOMS OF FOOD INTOLERANCE

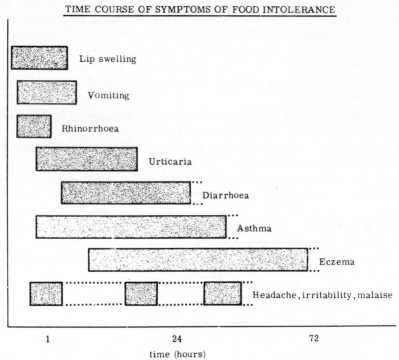

FIGURE 1   Food intolerance—symptoms and time course

Immediate and late reactions

The development of an immediate reaction within minutes of eating a certain food—swelling of the lips or tongue, rhinorrhoea, or such features as urticaria, asthma, or eczema—has been taken as providing presumptive evidence of an IgE-mediated reaction, although confusion with 'pseudo-allergic' disorders can occur (see Chapter 7). In allergic cases the total serum IgE level is usually raised and if an appropriate extract of the suspect food is available, a positive skin-prick test can often be elicited or a positive RAST obtained.

Where a patient's symptoms begin more than an hour after the food is ingested, or where they develop only after repeated exposure to the same food, evidence of an IgE reaction is less commonly found and it may be difficult to prove either the diagnosis or the presence of an immunological response of any kind. In such cases the most important first step is therefore to confirm by challenge methods that the reaction is food-related.

When food intolerance is confirmed—and especially if the symptoms are mainly abdominal—non-allergic causes should be considered, including lactose intolerance and disaccharidase deficiencies in general, peptic ulceration and gall stones, cystic fibrosis, low-grade intestinal infections, psychological illness, and the pharmacological effects of caffeine.

Where these are excluded, no fewer than 93 out of 100 patients in a recently analysed series were found to have suggestive evidence of an allergic reaction outside the gastrointestinal tract—such as asthma, eczema, urticaria, angioedema, rhinorrhoea, or anaphylaxis (Lessof *et al.*, 1980b). It has therefore been suggested that the diagnosis of food intolerance should be changed to food allergy only if there is clear clinical evidence of allergic features or a positive skin test or RAST. Even so, where the evidence of allergy is solely derived from clinical features such as urticaria, other explanations are possible—such as non-immunological histamine release or the pharmacological effect of food amines.

GASTROINTESTINAL EFFECTS

Apart from vomiting, diarrhoea, or abdominal pain, gastrointestinal effects in adults are similar to those seen in children and include abdominal distension, constipation, and a variety of symptoms associated with malabsorption or with protein-losing enteropathy. Anal pruritis is not uncommon in patients with diarrhoea, and exceptionally, a haemorrhagic proctitis can occur in patients with cow's milk intolerance (Buisseret *et al.*, 1978). Food-induced allergic symptoms also develop outside the intestinal tract and the smell of fish can provoke rhinitis or asthma in a sensitized subject, while local contact can provoke angioedema of the face or mouth. A delay in the onset of symptoms makes it likely that the route for sensitization is 'alimentary' rather than from the inhalation of odours or through surface contact. In such late-onset cases systemic symptoms may nevertheless occur, including acute anaphylactic reactions and shock, bronchial asthma, urticaria, and eczema.

The gastrointestinal symptoms which may be associated with allergic causes are summarized in Table 2. Although these have mainly been described in children they sometimes persist or even develop in adult life. Intestinal bleeding and iron deficiency anaemia can occur (Wilson *et al.*, 1964). In addition to diarrhoea, there may be hypoproteinaemia and eosinophilia, and when Waldmann and his colleagues (1967) described six children with these

TABLE 2   Gastrointestinal reactions to foods

1. Direct	Vomiting; diarrhoea; pain; bloating; constipation
2. Secondary	'Coeliac-like'; blood loss; iron deficiency; steatorrhoea; protein-losing enteropathy; eosinophilic gastroenteritis
3. Remote effects	Rhinorrhoea; serous otitis; asthma; eczema; urticaria; angioedema; anaphylaxis

changes, they noted an association with such other symptoms as rhinorrhoea, bronchial asthma, and eczema. A malabsorption syndrome due to cow's milk intolerance is probably much more common than has been realized, since Kuitunen and his colleagues were able to describe 54 cases (Kuitunen *et al.*, 1975).

Eosinophilic gastroenteritis

Eosinophilic gastroenteritis is an intriguing syndrome which can sometimes have an allergic cause—but perhaps not always. In this condition there is diffuse eosinophilic infiltration, usually in the pyloric region, associated with peripheral blood eosinophilia which is not due to intestinal parasites, vasculitis, neoplasm, or any other recognized local cause. Out of seven patients reported by Klein and his colleagues, together with a further 28 patients whose case reports were reviewed (Klein *et al.*, 1970), 16 had evidence of associated allergic disease elsewhere in the body, ranging from allergic rhinitis to angioedema, urticaria, and asthma. A reaction to specific foods may be difficult to recognize, and even when an exacerbation occurs after a food challenge, it does not follow that the elimination of that food from the diet will result in a remission of symptoms. While remissions have been reported in infancy and childhood when milk was excluded from the diet (Waldmann *et al.*, 1967), remissions have not necessarily been sustained without the addition of corticosteroids, which have provided the most consistently successful therapeutic approach. At least 18 of the patients reported and reviewed by Klein and his colleagues are known to have responded to corticosteroid treatment.

Most recorded cases of eosinophilic infiltration of the gastrointestinal tract have shown minimal mucosal infiltration and predominant involvement of deeper layers of the gut wall. Doubt has therefore been cast on the diagnostic validity of biopsy techniques which are capable of showing only superficial mucosal changes. However, although jejunal mucosal biopsy may occasionally allow diagnostic confusion with eosinophilic granuloma, polyarteritis, or gastric carcinoma, it seems probable that this technique will continue to provide the ancillary test on which this diagnosis is made—in selected patients who are known to have blood eosinophilia and who satisfy the other diagnostic criteria cited above. Where pyloric obstruction develops, and laparotomy can therefore be justified, it has nevertheless become apparent that the muscle layer and, indeed, the entire thickness of the bowel wall may be involved as the disease progresses. In some cases, subserosal changes are associated with ascites and there may be a marked eosinophilia in the ascitic fluid.

The identification of an associated food allergy, if it exists, can clearly be of the greatest importance, since it offers at least some hope that the process can be reversed. Reactions to food can be dangerous. Sudden death has been reported during a meal, associated with oedema of the gastric and duodenal lining (Salmon and Paulley, 1967).

It is now clear that it may not be sufficient to identify a single food which is capable of provoking a reaction. In a case reported by Nelson and his colleagues (1979)—that of a 9½-month-old white girl who presented with a protein-losing gastroenteropathy—parenteral feeding with an elemental diet led to a rapid fall in eosinophil count and a steady gain in weight. The blunted villi and submucosal oedema which had been noted on jejunal biopsy returned to normal, and at the end of 6 months on 'Vivonex' it was possible to resume a full diet except for milk, egg, and wheat products. Milk was not alone in provoking a relapse. Adding wheat to the diet led to a rise in blood eosinophils from 10 to 27 per cent of the total count.

From the therapeutic point of view, it is clear that the problem of eosinophilic gastroenteritis is far from solved. The use of intestinal challenge with suspected foods has been shown to be of value, however, so that an appropriate dietary regime can be devised (Caldwell et al., 1975). Even so, corticosteroids may be needed in addition to dietary restriction before the control of symptoms can be achieved.

Apart from the treatment of individual patients there is an additional reason for giving consideration to the multiple-food allergies which may be associated with eosinophilic gastroenteritis. There has been much controversy over the question of whether food allergies are ever serious enough to be life-threatening or to require treatment by elemental diets or within a controlled environment. Among the published cases of eosinophilic gastroenteritis there appear to be a very small number in which extreme allergies of this type may indeed exist.

Ulcerative colitis and haemorrhagic proctitis

Whereas the association between adult ulcerative colitis and food-allergic disease remains dubious, there is considerable evidence which suggests that among those patients who are diagnosed as having inflammatory bowel disease, there is a subgroup in whom allergic mechanisms play a considerable part. Rosenkrans and his colleagues (1980) studied 12 patients with isolated proctitis, none of whom had evidence of inflammation beyond the distal sigmoid colon. Histologically, there was a marked increase in IgE-containing cells in the lamina propria, and although allergy to a specific food was not identified, the eight patients with symptoms which were severe enough to require treatment all improved while taking oral disodium cromoglycate.

SKIN REACTIONS

Reactions to food are not confined to the gastrointestinal tract. Among the distant effects which occur, skin reactions are by no means uncommon.

In our own series of 100 patients with food intolerance, 22 were found to have urticaria or angioedema as a presenting feature, usually developing within 1 or 2 hours of taking the offending food. A further 37 had a history of eczema, which tended to develop more insidiously and to resolve more slowly. Other patients had noted—often in childhood—the development of macular or papular eruptions after eating ice cream, coloured sweets, or various other foods. Since these episodes rarely required medical treatment, they were recalled with difficulty and were easily omitted from the patient's medical records.

Urticaria

Urticaria is a physical sign rather than a disease, with a wide range of possible causes. These include:

(1) allergy, involving mast cell activation by IgE-mediated mechanisms;
(2) pharmacological effects, notably from amines in food;
(3) complement activation mediated by immune complex deposition (as in vasculitis);
(4) complement activation by other mechanisms, including intrinsic defects of the complement system (Chodirker *et al.*, 1979);
(5) non-immunological stimulation of mediator release—physical and cholinergic urticarias, provoked by such stimuli as cold, heat, light, pressure, vibration, exercise, or emotional stress (Dahl, 1981b).

Urticaria involves oedema and erythema of the skin, with a recurring accumulation of fluid in the dermis, apparently caused by a sudden increase in local vascular permeability. The lesions usually itch, change their form within minutes, and last from about ½ hour up to 72 hours or more. Where there are more diffuse oedematous reactions, involving deeper tissues, the term angioedema is used, and these two types of rash can alternate or coexist. Of the two, angioedema is the more severe, and if it involves the glottis, or is associated with anaphylaxis, it may be life-threatening.

Although the tissue fluid within an urticarial lesion cannot be studied directly, much can be inferred from the work of Kaplan *et al.* (1978) who raised suction blisters in the skin of patients with chronic urticaria and showed that the fluid contains more histamine than is usually found in control subjects. Furthermore, when an attempt is made to simulate the natural release of histamine by injecting it intradermally, local lesions of necrotizing vasculitis can be induced in these patients (Braverman and Yen, 1975; Gower *et al.*, 1976). Using this technique Dahl (1981b) has demonstrated the early deposition of C3 in the walls of dermal blood vessels, perhaps indicating that a local deposition of immune complexes has occurred.

It does not follow that histamine is the only mediator involved. The injection into the skin of a variety of mediators—serotonin, kinins, prostaglandins, and complement activation products (anaphylotoxins)—can all provoke urticarial reactions and can cause the necessary changes in vascular permeability. Since their release can be triggered both by immunological and non-immunological means, however, it cannot be assumed that all urticaria implies an immunological abnormality (Soter and Austen, 1976).

The changes which follow immediately after the release of mediators are evanascent, and a number of secondary consequences follow. The liberation of chemotactic factors plays a part in attracting eosinophils, neutrophils, and platelets to the area, which may at first serve to magnify the inflammatory effect. The cells which arrive in the area, particularly the eosinophils, may also help to limit the duration of the reaction, by inactivating such primary mediators as histamine and the leukotrienes (Wasserman *et al.*, 1975; Zeiger *et al.*, 1976). Histologically, the eventual appearances are those of a perivascular infiltrate, in which mononuclear cells and polymorphs are prominent. Occasionally, within such lesions, frank changes of necrotizing vasculitis may also be seen.

Foods, food additives, and urticaria

Urticaria is provoked by food more frequently in children than in adults. 44 per cent of children with urticaria were found by Halpern (1965) to have food intolerance, with symptoms which in the most severe cases included anaphylaxis and hypotension. The range of foods is similar to that mentioned in Table 1. As an example, yeast has taken a prominent place in recent studies

TABLE 3   Examples of food additives which can cause urticaria

Dyes
Tartrazine
Amaranth
New coccine, sunset yellow

Preservatives
Sodium benzoate
Sodium hydroxybenzoate
4-Hydroxybenzoic acid

Other additives
Fat antioxidants
Sodium nitrite
Sodium metabisulphite
Tyramine
Drugs (penicillin, tetracycline, quinine, menthol)

(James and Warin, 1971; Warin and Smith, 1976). It should be noted that the sources of yeast include not only bread, rice, sausage, alcoholic drinks, Marmite, and yeast tablets, but also *Candida* organisms in the gastrointestinal or genital tract. Cross-reactions to different foods may therefore require close analysis before it is concluded that the food is itself responsible for the patient's symptoms. This is especially true when synthetic food additives, such as azo-dyes and preservatives, are considered (see Table 3). Such additives are now thought to provoke urticaria in a high proportion of the more intractable cases (Lockey, 1971; August, 1980). In addition, most patients who react to dyes and preservatives also react to salicylates (Michaëlsson and Juhlin, 1973), including the amounts present in some fruits and vegetables.

Diagnosis of food-induced urticaria

It is often helpful if the patient can identify all foods taken within an hour or two of the development of urticaria, and a more extended dietary history can sometimes be of value. Recurrent attacks can, however, be difficult to analyse, partly because the phase of recovery following a severe episode of urticaria is often punctuated by the recurrence of minor episodes of skin rash, provoked by such non-specific factors as exercise, simple rubbing of the skin, other factors causing peripheral vasodilatation, or even the ingestion of other foods. The role of exercise is of particular relevance. Not only can it potentiate food-allergic urticaria (Maulitz *et al.*, 1979). Exercise has also been reported as provoking urticaria and even anaphylaxis, when there is no other evidence which might suggest an allergic cause (Sheffer and Austen, 1980). Emotion, stress, and fatigue have also been identified by some patients as factors which provoke a recurrence of a recently subsided allergic rash, although they have no effect once the underlying cause has been identified and treated. The contributory and sometimes confusing role of non-specific factors in allergic disease is, in fact, particularly well seen in urticaria (see Figure 2).

As with other types of food reaction, the use of simple elimination diets may be useful, followed by challenge tests which depend on choosing a series of suspect materials and giving them in sequence.

While food additives are frequently implicated in cases of chronic urticaria, their wide distribution among processed and 'convenience' foods may make it difficult to eliminate them from the modern diet. Attempts to provoke exacerbations of rash may therefore be useful, involving a daily series of challenge capsules which contain the most commonly involved substances — dyes such as tartrazine (5, 10, or 50 mg); powdered yeast tablets (3 BP tablets); 0.5 mg penicillin G or, as a control substance, 10 mg lactose. Sodium benzoate is included by some authors, but its role is doubtful. August (1980) has suggested that, where a single substance is to be tested at two or more dose levels, an interval of 1–1½ hours between doses is sufficient, and this has the

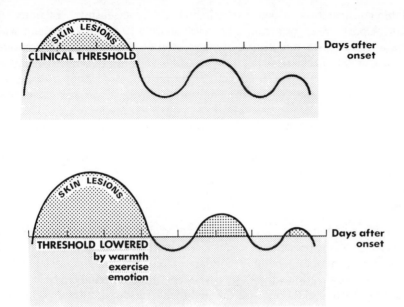

FIGURE 2   Urticaria — the potentiating effect of non-specific factors

advantage that a cumulative effect may sometimes be seen after successive challenges, whereas a simple challenge may fail to provoke urticaria. The challenge procedure may be disappointing in these controlled conditions, however, even in patients who have satisfied themselves that they have discovered a close relationship between the taking of a coloured food and the appearance of urticaria. For this failure, it is customary to blame psychological factors, although it would be as logical to invoke a lack of exercise or of some of the other potentiating factors mentioned above. In addition, it has been claimed that gross over-exposure may sometimes produce a temporary state of non-reactivity. Finally, the ease with which urticaria can be induced may itself wax and wane. This has led to an empirical approach which involves the banning of food additives for at least a month, whether or not a positive challenge test has been obtained. After a few weeks or months on an additive-free diet (Ros et al., 1976) a normal diet can often be tolerated without any sign of a return of urticaria.

Tests for IgE-mediated reactions

Because of the many different physiological pathways which can lead to urticaria, the presence of this symptom in patients with specific food intolerance is no proof that an immediate type of hypersensitivity is involved. A positive skin-prick test or RAST with the appropriate food provides the best available confirmatory evidence that immediate hypersensitive reactions are present. A positive test was found, however, in only 10 out of 22 patients with food-induced angioedema or urticaria (Lessof et al., 1980b). This leaves some doubt about the mechanism involved in those with negative tests, many of whom may be reacting to food amines or histamine-releasing substances. Even where an immunological mechanism is suspected, negative tests may either indicate that IgE is not involved or that the test methods are inadequate (as may be the case where food additives are concerned). Certainly, IgE mechanisms, by themselves, can no longer explain all the observed clinical features, even in the presence of asthma or other symptoms which suggest an atopic reaction.

Eczema

Eczema is an itching red rash which often affects the flexures and is also characterized by the presence of scaling, vesiculation, exudation, and crusting. Added to this, there may be the secondary effects of scratching and bacterial infection. An association with atopy is very common, especially in cases which originate in early childhood, and the presence of asthma, allergic rhinitis, a family history of atopy, or a high serum IgE level frequently provide further evidence to support an allergic origin (Barnetson and Merrett, 1980).

Histologically, the most characteristic changes are an intracellular oedema and vacuolation of keratinocytes which is seen in the epidermis (Dahl, 1981b). In the dermis, an inflammatory infiltrate is present, consisting mainly of mononuclear cells in well-established lesions but including some basophils, especially in the developing stages of eczematous lesions which are induced by patch testing (Mitchell et al., 1982).

Despite its association with high IgE levels and other features of immediate hypersensitivity, the slow evolution of eczema and the eventual histological appearances are more suggestive of delayed hypersensitivity than of an immediate allergic response. The early presence of basophils may provide the key to this apparent contradiction, and the delayed onset might be compatible with the time-scale of cutaneous basophil hypersensitivity, which is known to involve the slow accumulation of basophils in the tissues. When the basophils degranulate and release their enzymes, there is a local increase in vascular permeability (Askenase et al., 1981). This could help to provoke the added features of a classical, delayed hypersensitivity reaction, which are so conspicuous in the fully developed lesions. The evidence thus suggests that more than one immunological mechanism is involved.

Food allergy and eczema

In children, at least, food allergy is a very potent provoking factor, and Goldman et al. (1963) was able to demonstrate an exacerbation of eczema after milk challenge in 31 out of 37 children whose parents had already made the observation that cow's milk exacerbated their symptom. Conversely, a restricted diet may be beneficial. When egg was excluded from the diet of children who had both atopic eczema and a positive skin-prick test to egg, Meara (1965) noted an improvement in 11 out of 29 cases. The relationship was not a simple one, since the re-introduction of egg was more likely to cause urticaria (eight cases) than eczema (two cases). The adverse effect of egg was nevertheless established in these cases. Atherton and his colleagues (1978) also found that 14 out of 20 children with eczema improved on a diet which excluded both cow's milk and eggs. In the same study, only one child improved on an unrestricted diet.

The response to elimination diets in adults is less dependable, even in cases with a positive skin-prick test and a clear history of food-induced exacerbations of the skin condition.

ASTHMA

Food-induced asthma is also well recognized, and up to 17 per cent of asthmatic patients believe that particular foods can provoke an asthmatic attack (Burr, 1980). However, it is not always clear whether it is provoked by inhaled odours or by the alimentary route. The smell of fish may be sufficient to induce an immediate asthmatic attack in fish-allergic individuals, and there are a number of other examples of this kind. There are, on the other hand, many cases in which the ingestion of food may be followed by an asthmatic attack one or two hours later, when it is less likely that the inhalational route is involved. Nor is it only delayed-onset asthma which can be provoked via the gastrointestinal tract. During blind challenge studies through a nasogastric tube, attacks of asthma may be induced within a period of minutes (J. B. Anderson, personal communication), again suggesting that even the immediate development of bronchospasm is not always triggered by the inhalational route.

The route by which foods can trigger an asthmatic attack can thus vary from one patient to another and it can also vary with different foods. Alcoholic drinks can provoke asthma when taken by mouth, whereas alcohol contained in fumes or given by intravenous injection is said to be less likely to do so (Gong et al., 1981). In some cases it is the congeners of alcohol which have been thought to cause bronchospasm, and the suspect substances include yeasts, fungi, and flavouring or colouring agents. The histamine which is found in red and white wine has also been invoked and so has the potent, histamine-releasing effect of the aldehyde ethanal (see Chapter 7). Particular beverages can provoke asthmatic attacks when the equivalent amount of ethyl alcohol fails to do so (Breslin et al., 1973); but in such cases there is often no evidence of atopy, and skin tests with yeasts and wine extracts tend to be negative. It may nevertheless be possible to prevent the reaction by pretreatment with inhaled cromoglycate.

This is not the whole story. Although unadulterated ethyl alcohol usually increases the vital capacity of asthmatic subjects (Herxheimer and Stresemann, 1963) it, too, can cause bronchospasm in a few patients. In a detailed study of one such case Gong and his colleagues (1981) noted first that the response to inhaled histamine indicated a marked bronchial hyperreactivity, and then that a partial inhibition of the asthmatic response could be achieved by such diverse agents as atropine, chlorpheniramine, and cyproheptadine. Since none of these inhibitors was totally effective it was argued that several mediators may be involved and that cholinergic nervous pathways, histamine, and serotonin all contribute. In this study sodium cromoglycate, whether given by inhalation or as a 200 mg oral dose, failed to prevent the asthmatic response. It was therefore suggested that the release of mediators from gastrointestinal sites could not provide an adequate explanation for this phenomenon. This conclusion may need to be modified, however, in view of the observation (Dahl, 1981a) that larger doses of cromoglycate may be of prophylactic value in some cases of food-induced asthma.

The absence of obvious evidence of associated classical allergic phenomena may not be confined to those with alcohol-induced asthma. Most patients with food-induced asthma have high IgE levels and often have a positive skin test or RAST to the appropriate food, but a sub-group has been described with 'low-IgE asthma' and negative tests. Five patients with milk intolerance had IgE levels below 40 units/ml, negative skin tests, and RASTs, and no evidence of IgG antibodies (Lessof *et al.*, 1980b). They nevertheless had asthmatic reactions which sometimes developed an hour or more after drinking milk. This provides a further example of 'alimentary' asthma and again cannot be explained as a response to inhaled allergens or to a non-specific bronchial response to irritant gases, histamine, or hyperventilation. The mechanism, however, remains unclear. If asthma is triggered by the systemic route, after the absorption of milk proteins from the gut, it is a reasonable hypothesis that this could be due to mediators released in the gastrointestinal tract (Lessof *et al.*, 1979). It has also been suggested that these symptoms may be triggered by circulating, food antigen-containing immune complexes, which might either contain IgG or IgE antibodies — or both (Brostoff *et al.*, 1979).

Other pulmonary syndromes

It remains to be seen whether asthma will prove to be the only food-allergic reaction to affect the lungs in adults. A syndrome of chronic respiratory disease has also been described in children with hypersensitivity to cow's milk, which may be followed by pulmonary haemosiderosis (Heiner *et al.*, 1962; Lee *et al.*, 1978; Bahna and Heiner, 1980). There is no direct evidence of a similar effect in adults, but patients with gluten enteropathy and an abnormal intestinal mucosa not infrequently become sensitized and develop antibodies to a component of hen egg yolk (Faux *et al.*, 1978). Bearing this in mind, it is intriguing to note that patients with gluten enteropathy also seem to be particularly prone to develop bird fancier's lung (Berrill *et al.*, 1979).

Diagnosis of food-induced asthma

When an asthmatic response to ingested food antigens is suspected, serial estimations of peak flow values should be recorded by the patient at home over a period of days or weeks, and correlated with a diary of food intake (Wraith, 1980). At its simplest, this may disclose that a drop in peak flow value follows, regularly and predictably, the intake of an individual food. More difficult to analyse are those insidious and prolonged episodes of bronchospasm which appear to relate to more than one food and to be influenced, in addition, by precipitating factors such as exercise, cold weather, or contact with other allergens, including animal proteins and dust mites. The additive effects of these factors can be considerable, as in the well-documented case of the athlete who had anaphylactic reactions if he ate shellfish and then went for a long-distance run (Maulitz *et al.*, 1979).

In some food-allergic subjects, asthma develops only at the end of a prolonged period, after repeated challenge with the appropriate food. In such cases recovery is also likely to be slow, and Wraith has noted that symptoms such as intermittent diarrhoea, pains in the joints, and depression can further confuse the clinical story. The cumulative effects of repeated 'challenge' may, perhaps, explain some of these features—notably the drawn-out time-scale. Such a time-scale is reminiscent of that seen in occupational asthma after the repeated inhalation of industrial chemicals. The development of joint pains, however, suggests that other mechanisms—perhaps including immune complex reactions—may be involved.

In following a diagnostic suspicion that is directed against a particular food, it may be sufficient to give a simple elimination diet over a period of 2 or 3 weeks. If symptoms subside during this period, it then becomes possible to carry out a formal challenge test. Often, however, there is no clear response to a simplified diet and, despite the patient's own suspicions, the history remains inconclusive or suggests that more than one food is involved. Since the next steps involve the more severe food-restriction regimes, the justification for further investigation may need to be considered. In such cases, circumstantial supporting evidence can be provided by a history of food sensitivity and eczema in childhood, by a positive skin-prick test or RAST, or in some cases by the patient's assertion that repeated experiments with different dietary regimes have led to remissions and exacerbations.

If it is decided to pursue the diagnosis of food-induced asthma, some physicians prefer to use an elimination diet as has been outlined earlier in this chapter. Others proceed directly to the fasting regime of Wraith, with 4 or 5 days as an inpatient, taking either water only, or a synthetic food. As with other food-induced symptoms, there may be difficulty in separating a directly induced food allergy from a reaction to artificial colouring agents such as azo-dyes which are found not only in foods but in the coloured coating of antihistamines and other drugs.

RHINORRHOEA

Rhinorrhoea is also frequently mentioned by patients, often as a reaction to the smell of the relevant food. Stimulation by the inhalational route does not always seem to be involved, however, since rhinitis has been described in double-blind studies, in which milk is introduced into the stomach through a nasogastric tube (Bock *et al.*, 1978).

JOINT PAINS AND ARTHRITIS

Wraith (1980) is not alone in reporting joint pains as a manifestation of food sensitivity. Parke and Hughes (1981) have given details of a patient with a long-standing, seronegative rheumatoid arthritis who had a passion for cheese and lost her symptoms on a diet which was free of dairy produce. On repeated occasions, within 12 hours of re-introducing cheese she not only relapsed clinically—with pain, stiffness, and objective changes in joint measurements—but also developed a leukocytosis, a change in the concentration of circulating immune complexes, and a positive RAST for IgE antibodies to milk and cheese protein.

Parke and Hughes made no claims about the mechanism by which cheese protein provoked an exacerbation of symptoms in their patients. They made one other observation, however, which may be relevant. When heat-damaged red cells were injected intravenously, it was shown that the rate of clearance of these cells was normal before the challenge test. However, the rate of clearance of these cells was considerably prolonged at the end of the test and remained so 12 days later. If, as seems likely, this indicated a defect of reticuloendothelial function (Elkon *et al.*, 1980) it seems possible that some of this patient's symptoms may have been related to a failure to clear immune complexes containing milk and cheese protein.

NEPHROTIC SYNDROME

A number of other unusual symptoms have occasionally been related to food hypersensitivity. Sandberg and his colleagues (1977) described six patients who each had a steroid-responsive nephrotic syndrome, in whom cow's milk was shown to provoke a relapse, and withdrawal of milk led to a partial or complete remission. Interestingly, there was an associated asthma or eczema in all but one case. While food allergy may not be a common cause of the nephrotic syndrome in childhood, extremely high serum IgE levels (over 1500 IU/ml) have been reported in 10 out of 84 children with a steroid-sensitive nephrotic syndrome (Meadow et al., 1981). Both positive skin tests to foods and positive basophil degranulation tests have also been reported in a small number of cases (Pirotzky et al., 1982). This suggests that a more intensive search may be required, if food-allergic and other treatable causes of the nephrotic syndrome are to be identified.

THROMBOCYTOPAENIA

It appears that cow's milk may provoke episodes of thrombocytopaenia, notably in cases with congenital absence of the radius in which there is presumably another underlying cause for this condition (Whitfield and Barr, 1976). A recently reported case of an adult with severe thrombocytopaenia, which was reversed on a milk-free diet (Caffrey et al., 1981), has shown the difficulty in establishing both the diagnosis and the mechanism in such complex cases.

PSYCHIATRIC SYMPTOMS

Among the most controversial claims that have been made in relationship to food intolerance are the claims that much psychiatric health and depression is food-induced (see Chapter 2). While many of the claims which have been made do not stand up to critical examination, it is widely believed that mental changes and psychiatric ill-health can be a prominent feature of coeliac disease (see Chapter 9). In addition, there have been numerous instances (Buisseret, 1978) in which, on a satisfactorily restricted diet, the irritability and behaviour disorders of a milk-allergic child have disappeared together with asthma, eczema, and other manifestations which have the clinical hallmarks of allergy. If it is therefore accepted that mental changes can accompany gluten enteropathy, and that a change in behaviour can follow the treatment of food allergy in a child, it seems illogical to deny that food allergy may be a cause of psychiatric ill-health in adults. This diagnosis remains controversial, however, mainly because the label of 'food-allergic' psychiatric illness is often used without reference to any diagnostic criteria and without evidence of any associated allergic manifestations or immunological abnormality. Since overt psychiatric symptoms were not an obtrusive feature of 100 consecutive cases of confirmed food intolerance (Lessof et al., 1980b), it may be particularly important to distinguish patients with food fads and obsessional neuroses from those who have a food-allergic disorder. It is in this group of patients that the results of food-elimination diets and blind challenge methods need to be most scrupulously applied.

MANAGEMENT

The steps which are necessary for the identification and restriction of major food allergens have been discussed above. Elimination of a particular suspect food—for example, strawberries or shellfish—presents no problems, but progression to the more strict elimination diets can cause difficulties. For the more restricted regimes, a dietitian's help may be needed to ensure the adequacy of protein, calories, calcium, and vitamins.

TABLE 4   Simple exclusion diet*

Permitted	Major exclusions
Lamb or mutton	Other meat and poultry. Fish
Gluten-free bread, rice (and Rice Krispies)	Other bread, cakes, biscuits, pasta, cereals
Tomor margarine	Milk, butter and dairy products. Eggs
Fresh fruit and vegetables	Strawberries, nuts, preserves, and commercially frozen food
Tea, coffee, sugar, fresh fruit juice	Wines and spirits
Barley sugar	Confectionery
Olive oil	

*Modified from a diet employed by the Department of Dietetics, Northwick Park Hospital (Denman, 1980).

The first objective of an exclusion diet is to eliminate those foods which are the most frequent cause of reactions and, at the same time, to provide a regime which can be managed by the patient without constant expert supervision. The foods which are the most frequent cause of problems include milk, egg, fish, nuts, spices, and artificially coloured or preserved foods of various kinds. The diet which is detailed in Table 4 contains easily available ingredients, with the possible exception of gluten-free bread which can be omitted. It has the practical advantage that it can be followed without difficulty on an outpatient basis for a period of a week or two—or longer if necessary. If the patient's symptoms have cleared at the end of an initial period of dieting, it can be assumed that the items of food contained in the diet are not a cause of symptoms. Once a diet has been found on which the patient can remain well, that diet can be continued and a succession of new foods added, each one being taken in reasonably large quantities for a period of a few days. If symptoms do not return, the presumption is made that the new food is safe, but if the symptoms do come back, the most recently added food is suspected as the cause and more formal challenge tests can then be initiated.

Should the initial diet fail to relieve symptoms, and if the evidence of food intolerance is sufficient to justify further efforts, it may seem reasonable to continue with the same type of diet, now modified by removing one or two suspect foods for a further week or two. The alternatives are to try to change a few ingredients in the empirical diet (see Table 5), or to proceed to a much more basic dietary regime on an inpatient basis, initially giving water or an elemental diet of the 'Vivonex' type while monitoring peak flow measurements

TABLE 5   Simple exclusion diet — alternative ingredients

		Substituting for
Meat	Beef or chicken	Lamb or mutton
Cereal	Rye crispbread Maize (and cornflakes) Tapioca	Gluten-free bread Rice
Vegetables	Continue carrots, lettuce, potatoes	Exclude beans, peas, soy
Fruits	Continue prunes, pears, apricots, peaches, pineapples	Exclude citrus fruits and apples
Drinks	Water	Tea, coffee, fruit juice
Cooking oil	Corn oil Sunflower seed oil Cottonseed oil	Olive oil
Miscellaneous	Corn syrup	Sugar

and other indicators which might provide an objective assessment of asthmatic or other severe symptoms. In general, the patients who are investigated in this way will have clear evidence of a severe and classical allergic disorder associated, for example, with asthma or eczema. Occasionally, however, the provisional clinical diagnosis will be one of psychiatric ill-health and the indication for investigation may be the need to demonstrate, to the satisfaction of all concerned, whether a patient's self-diagnosis of 'food allergy' can be sustained or not.

Drug treatment

Where drugs are needed — and especially when reactions to artificial colours or preservatives are suspected — the use of coloured antihistamines or other pills should be avoided, as should syrup preparations, which are likely to contain both artificial colouring and preservative. Antihistamines which are not coloured include bromphenyramine (Dimotane), mebhydrolin (Fabihistin), hydroxyzine (Atarax), azatadine (Optimine), and terfenadine (Triludan), a recently released preparation which appears to be remarkably free of sedative effects.

Anti-inflammatory drugs

Aspirin and other non-steroidal anti-inflammatory drugs have been used with some success in the symptomatic treatment of diarrhoea and other gastro-intestinal reactions (Buisseret *et al.*, 1978). Since prostaglandin synthetase inhibitors have also been found to relieve other types of diarrhoea, the effect is presumably non-specific.

Sodium cromoglycate

As has been mentioned above, both oral and inhaled sodium cromoglycate have been used for their prophylactic effect in patients with IgE-mediated food allergy or sensitivity to acetyl salicylic acid (Dahl, 1981a). When patients were treated with 400 mg sodium cromoglycate on a total of five occasions over a 24-hour period, this was shown to prevent an asthmatic response to food challenge, whereas inhalations of 40 mg sodium cromoglycate had no effect. However, neither form of sodium cromoglycate was effective against aspirin-induced asthma. A large number of similar studies have now been carried out and have been reviewed by Edwards (1980).

The dose–response pattern for sodium cromoglycate is still not fully understood. It remains to be seen whether food-induced symptoms which fail to respond to smaller doses of this drug may nevertheless respond to a different drug regime. Wraith *et al.* (1979) have used a three or four times daily regime giving the drug before meals in total daily doses of 300–2000 mg in adults and have claimed excellent results. Formulation may be important, since Vaz *et al.* (1978), using a weak aqueous solution which was swilled round the mouth and then swallowed, found that 100–400 mg provided an effective daily dose. Basomba and his colleagues (1977), using cromoglycate tablets, also reported a satisfactory clinical response, but only in a dose range which was similar to that reported by Wraith.

REFERENCES

Aalberse, R. C., Koshte, V., and Clemens, J. G. S. (1981). Cross-reactions between vegetable foods, pollen and bee venom due to IgE antibodies to a ubiquitous carbohydrate determinant. *Int. Arch. Allergy Appl. Immunol.*, **66** (suppl.), 259–60.
Aas, K., and Lundkvist, U. (1973). The radioallergosorbent test with a purified allergen from codfish. *Clin. Allergy*, **3**, 255–61.
Ament, M. D., and Rubin, C. E. (1972). Soy protein—another cause of flat intestinal lesion. *Gastroenterology*, **62**, 227–34.

Anand, B. S., Piris, J., Jerrome, D. W., Offord, R. E., and Truelove, S. C. (1981). The timing of histological damage following a single challenge with gluten in treated coeliac disease. *Quart. J. Med.*, **197**, 83–94.

Askenase, P. W., Mitchell, E. B., and Brown, S. J. (1981). Cutaneous basophil hypersensitivity: mediation, regulaton and effector function. In: *Factors Affecting Sensitivity to Allergens in Atopic Disease* (ed. H. O. J. Collier). Dome/Hollister-Stier, Stoke Poges, pp.43–5.

Atherton, D. J., Sewell, M., Soothill, J. F., Wells, R. S., and Chilvers, C. E. C. (1978). A double-blind controlled crossover trial of an antigen-avoidance diet in atopic eczema. *Lancet*, **1**, 401–3.

August, P. J. (1980). Urticaria. In: *Proceedings of the First Food Allergy Workshop* (ed. R. R. A. Coombs). Medical Education Services, Oxford, pp.76–81.

Bahna, S. L., and Heiner, D. C. (1980). *Allergies to Milk.* Grune & Stratton, New York.

Barnetson, R. StC., and Merrett, T. G. (1980). Atopic eczema. In: *Proceedings of the First Food Allergy Workshop* (ed. R. R. A. Coombs). Medical Education Services, Oxford, pp.69–75.

Basomba, A., Campos, A., Villalmanzo, I. G., and Pelacz, A. (1977). The effect of sodium cromoglycate in patients with food allergies. *Acta Allergy*, **32** (suppl. 13), 96.

Berrens, L., van Dijk, A. G., and Weemaes, C. M. R. (1981). Complement consumption in egg white and fish sensitivity. *Clin. Allergy.*, **11**, 101–9.

Berrill, W. T., Eade, O. E., Fitzpatrick, P. F., Hyde, I., MacLeod, W. M., and Wright, R. (1975). Bird-fancier's lung and jejunal villous atrophy. *Lancet*, **2**, 1006.

Blumenthal, I., Kelleher, J., and Littlewood, J. M. (1981). Recurrent abdominal pain and lactose intolerance in childhood. *Br. Med. J.*, **282**, 2013–14.

Bock, S. A., Buckley, J., Holst, A., and May, C. D. (1977). Proper use of skin tests with food extracts. *Clin. Allergy*, **7**, 375–83.

Bock, S. A., Lee, W.-Y., Remigio, L. K., and May, C. D. (1978). Studies of hypersensitivity reactions to foods in infants and children. *J. Allergy Clin. Immunol.*, **62**, 327–34.

Braverman, I. M., and Yen, A. (1975). Demonstration of immune complexes in spontaneous and histamine induced lesions and in normal skin of patients with leukocytoclastic angiitis. *J. Invest. Dermatol.*, **64**, 105–12.

Breslin, A. B. X., Hendrick, D. J., and Pepys, J. (1973). Effect of disodium cromoglycate on asthmatic reactions to alcoholic beverages. *Clin. Allergy*, **3**, 71–82.

Brostoff, J., Carini, C., Wraith, D. G., and Johns, P. (1979). Production of IgE complexes by allergen challenge in atopic patients and the effect of sodium cromoglycate. *Lancet*, **1**, 1268–70.

Buisseret, P. D. (1978). Common manifestations of cow's milk allergy in children. *Lancet*, **1**, 304–5.

Buisseret, P. D., Youlten, L. J. F., Heinzelman, D. I., and Lessof, M. H. (1978). Prostaglandin-synthesis inhibitors in prophylaxis of food intolerance. *Lancet*, **1**, 906–8.

Burr, M. L. (1980). Epidemiology. In: *Proceedings of the First Food Allergy Workshop* (ed. R. R. A. Coombs). Medical Education Service, Oxford, pp.9–12.

Caffrey, E. A., Sladen, G. E., Isaacs, P. E. T., and Clark, K. G. A. (1981). Thrombocytopenia caused by cow's milk. *Lancet*, **2**, 316.

Cairns, S. A., London, A., and Mallick, N. P. (1981). Circulating immune complexes following food: delayed clearance in idiopathic glomerulonephritis. *Clin. Exp. Immunol.*, **40**, 273–82.

Caldwell, J. H., Tennenbaum, J. I., and Bronstein, H. A. (1975). Serum IgE in eosinophilic gastroenteritis. *N. Engl. J. Med.*, **292**, 1388–90.

Chodirker, W. B., Bauman, W., and Komar, R. R. (1979). Immunological parameters and α_1-antitrypsin in chronic urticaria. *Clin. Allergy*, **9**, 201–10.

Cooper, B. T., Holmes, G. K. T., Ferguson, R., Thompson, R. A., Allan, R. N., and Cooke, W. T. (1980). Gluten-sensitive diarrhoea without evidence of coeliac disease. *Gastroenterology*, **79**, 801–6.

Cornell, H. J., and Rolles, C. J. (1978). Further evidence of a primary mucosal defect in coeliac disease. *Gut*, **19**, 253–9.

Dahl, R. (1981a). Oral and inhaled sodium cromoglycate in challenge tests with food allergens or acetylsalicylic acid. *Allergy*, **36**, 161–5.

Dahl, M. G. C. (1981b). Allergy and the skin. In: *Immunological and Clinical Aspects of Allergy* (ed. M. H. Lessof). MTP Press, Lancaster, pp.179–215.

Dannaeus, A., Inganäs, M., Johansson, S. G. O., and Foucard, T. (1979). Intestinal uptake of ovalbumin in malabsorption and food allergy in relation to serum IgG antibody and orally administered sodium cromoglycate. *Clin. Allergy*, **9**, 263–70.

Denman, A. M. (1980). Diagnostic methods and criteria. In: *Proceedings of the First Food Allergy Workshop* (ed. R. R. A. Coombs). Medical Education Services, Oxford, pp.47–55.

Edwards, A. M. (1980). Drug management. In: *Proceedings of the First Food Allergy Workshop* (ed. R. R. A. Coombs). Medical Education Services, Oxford, pp.95–101.

Elkon, K. B., Sewell, J. R., Ryan, P. F. J., and Hughes, G. R. V. (1980). Splenic function in non-renal systemic lupus erythematosus. *Am. J. Med.*, **69**, 80–91.

Eriksson, N. E. (1977). Diagnosis of reaginic allergy with house dust, animal dander and pollen allergens in adult patients. *Int. Arch. Allergy*, **53**, 341–8.

Faux, J. A., Hendrick, D. J., and Anand, B. S. (1978). Precipitins to different avian serum antigens in bird fancier's lung and coeliac disease. *Clin. Allergy*, **8**, 101–8.

Finn, R., and Cohen, H. N. (1978). Food allergy: fact or fiction? *Lancet*, **1**, 426–8.

Frick, O. L., German, D. F., and Mills, J. (1979). Development of allergy in children I. Association with virus infections. *J. Allergy Clin. Immunol.*, **63**, 228–41.

Fries, J. H. (1947). Milk allergy—diagnostic aspects and the role of milk substitutes. *J. Am. Med. Assoc.*, **165**, 1542–3.

Fries, J. H. (1971). Studies on the allergenicity of soy bean. *Ann. Allergy*, **29**, 1–5.

Fries, J. H. (1981). Food allergy: current concerns. *Ann. Allergy*, **46**, 260–3.

Goldman, A. S., Anderson, D. W., Sellers, W. A., Saperstein, S., Kniker, W. J., Halpern, S. R. *et al.* (1963). Milk allergy—I. Oral challenge with milk and isolated milk proteins in allergic children. *Pediatrics*, **32**, 425–43.

Goldman, A. S., and Heiner, D. C. (1977). Clinical aspects of food sensitivity. Diagnosis and management of cow's milk sensitivity. *Pediatr. Clin. N. Am.*, **24**, 133–5.

Gong, H., Tashkin, D. P., and Calvarese, B. M. (1981). Alcohol-induced bronchospasm in an asthmatic patient. *Chest*, **80**, 167–73.

Gower, R. G., Sams, W. M., Thorne, G., and Claman, H. N. (1976). Immune complex deposition in leukocytoclastic vasculitis. *J. Invest. Dermatol.*, **66**, 271.

Gwynn, C. M., Ingram, J., Almousawi, T., and Stanworth, D. R. (1982). Bronchial provocation tests in atopic patients with allergen-specific IgG4 antibodies. *Lancet*, **1**, 254–6.

Halpern, S. R. (1965). Chronic hives in children. An analysis of 75 cases. *Ann. Allergy*, **23**, 589–93.

Harnett, J. C., Spector, S. L., and Farr, R. S. (1978). Aspirin idiosyncrasy, asthma and urticaria. In: *Allergy: Principles and Practice* (eds E. Middleton, C. E. Reed and E. F. Ellis). C. V. Mosby, St Louis, pp.1002–22.

Heiner, D. C., Sears, J. W., and Kniker, W. T. (1962). Multiple precipitins to cow's milk in chronic respiratory disease. *Am. J. Dis. Child.*, **103**, 634–54.

Herxheimer, H., and Stresemann, E. (1963). Ethanol and lung function in bronchial asthma. *Arch. Internat. de Pharmacol. Therapie*, **144**, 310.

Hoffman, D. R., Day, E. D., and Miller, J. S. (1981). The major heat stable allergen of shrimp. *Ann. Allergy*, **47**, 17-22.

Jackson, P. G., Lessof, M. H., Baker, R. W. R., Ferrett, J., and MacDonald, D. M. (1981). Intestinal permeability in patients with eczema and food allergy. *Lancet*, **1**, 1285-7.

James, J., and Warin, R. P. (1971). An assessment of the role of *Candida albicans* and food yeasts in chronic urticaria. *Br. J. Dermatol.*, **84**, 227-37.

Kalish, G. H. (1981). Headaches after red wine. *Lancet*, **1**, 1263.

Kaplan, A. P., Horakova, Z., and Katz, S. I. (1978). Assessment of tissue fluid histamine levels in patients with urticaria. *J. Allergy Clin. Immunol.*, **61**, 350-4.

Kaufman, H. (1981). Headaches after red wine. *Lancet*, **1**, 1263.

Klein, N. C., Hargrove, R. L., Slesinger, M. H., and Jeffries, G. H. (1970). Eosinophilic gastroenteritis. *Medicine (Baltimore)*, **49**, 299-319.

Kuitunen, P., Visakorpi, J. K., Savilahti, E., and Pelkonen, P. (1975). Malabsorption syndrome with cow's milk intolerance. Clinical findings and course in 54 cases. *Arch. Dis. Child.*, **50**, 351-6.

Kwok, R. H. M. (1968). Chinese restaurant syndrome. *N. Engl. J. Med.*, **278**, 796.

Lee, S. K., Kniker, W. T., Cook, C. D., and Heiner, D. C. (1978). Cow's milk-induced pulmonary disease in children. In: *Advances in Pediatrics*. (ed. L. A. Barness). Year Book Medical Publishers, Chicago, pp.39-57.

Lessof, M. H. (1981). *Immunological and Clinical Aspects of Allergy*. MTP Press, Lancaster.

Lessof, M. H., Buisseret, P. D., Merrett, T. G., Merrett, J., Wraith, D. G., and Youlten, L. J. F. (1979). Mechanisms involving prostaglandins in food intolerance. In: *The Mast Cell: Its Role in Health and Disease* (ed. J. Pepys and A. M. Edwards). Pitman Medical, Tunbridge Wells, pp.406-10.

Lessof, M. H., Buisseret, P. D., Merrett, J., Merrett, T. G., and Wraith, D. G. (1980a). Assessing the value of skin prick tests. *Clin. Allergy*, **10**, 115-20.

Lessof, M. H., Wraith, D. G., Merrett, T. G., Merrett, J., and Buisseret, P. D. (1980b). Food allergy and intolerance in 100 patients—local and systemic effects. *Quart. J. Med.*, **195**, 259-71.

Lockey, S. D. (1971). Reactions to hidden agents in foods, beverages and drugs. *Ann. Allergy*, **29**, 461-9.

Lockey, S. D. (1972). Sensitizing properties of food additives and other commercial products. *Ann. Allergy*, **30**, 638-42.

Maulitz, R. M., Pratt, D. S., and Schocket, A. L. (1979). Exercise-induced anaphylactic reaction to shellfish. *J. Allergy Clin. Immunol.*, **63**, 433-4.

Meadow, S. R., Sarsfield, J. K., Scott, D. G., and Rajah, S. M. (1981). Steroid-responsive nephrotic syndrome and allergy: immunological studies. *Arch. Dis. Child.*, **56**, 517-24.

Meara, R. H. (1965). Skin reactions in atopic eczema. *Br. J. Dermatol.*, **67**, 60-4.

Michaëlsson, G., and Juhlin, L. (1973). Urticaria induced by preservatives and dye additives in food and drugs. *Br. J. Dermatol.*, **88**, 525-32.

Mitchell, E. B., Crow, J., Chapman, M. D., Jouhal, S. S., Pope, F. M., and Platts-Mills, T. A. E. (1982). Basophils in allergen-induced patch test sites in atopic dermatitis. *Lancet*, **1**, 127-30.

Moneret-Vautrin, D. A. (1979). Food pseudo-allergy. In: *The Mast Cell. Its Role in Health and Disease* (eds J. Pepys and A. M. Edwards). Pitman Medical, Tunbridge Wells, pp.431-7.

Mygind, N., and Thomsen, J. (1981). Allergic disorders of the ear. In: *Immunological and Clinical Aspects of Allergy* (ed. M. H. Lessof). MTP Press, Lancaster, pp.357–63.

Nelson, T. L., Klein, G. L., and Galant, S. P. (1979). Severe eosinophilic gastro-enteritis successfully treated with an elemental diet. *J. Allergy Clin. Immunol.*, **63**, 198.

Paganelli, R., Levinsky, R. J., Brostoff, J., and Wraith, D. G. (1979). Immune complexes containing food proteins in normal and atopic subjects after oral challenge and effect of sodium cromoglycate on antigen absorption. *Lancet*, **1**, 1270–2.

Paganelli, R., Levinsky, R. J., and Atherton, D. J. (1981). Detection of specific antigen within circulating immune complexes: validation of the assay and its application to food antigen–antibody complexes formed in health and food-allergic subjects. *Clin. Exp. Immunol.*, **46**, 44–53.

Parish, W. E. (1978). Evidence for human IgG antibodies anaphylactically sensitizing man. In: *Immediate hypersensitivity; Modern Concepts and Developments* (ed. M. K. Bach). Marcel Dekker, New York, pp.277–99.

Parke, A. L., and Hughes, G. R. V. (1981). Rheumatoid arthritis and food: a case study. *Br. Med. J.*, **282**, 2027–9.

Pepys, J., Parish, W. E., Stenius-Aarniala, B., and Wide, L. (1979). Clinical correlations between long-term (IgE) and short-term (IgG S-TS) anaphylactic antibodies in atopic and 'non-atopic' subjects with respiratory allergic disease. *Clin. Allergy*, **9**, 645–58.

Pirotzky, E., Hieblot, C., Benveniste, J., Laurent, J., Lagrue, G., and Noirot, C. (1982). Basophil sensitisation in idiopathic nephrotic syndrome. *Lancet*, **1**, 358–60.

Proceedings of the First Food Allergy Workshop (1980). (ed. R. R. A. Coombs.) Medical Education Services, Oxford.

Ros, A. M., Juhlin, L., and Michaélsson, G. (1976). A follow-up study of patients with recurrent urticaria and hypersensitivity to aspirin, benzoates and azo dyes. *Br. J. Dermatol.*, **95**, 19–24.

Rosenkrans, P. C. M., Meijer, C. J. L. M., van der Wal, A. M., and Lindeman, D. (1980). Allergic proctitis, a clinical and immunopathological entity. *Gut*, **21**, 1017–23.

Salmon, P. R., and Paulley, J. W. (1967). Eosinophilic granuloma of the gastro-intestinal tract. *Gut*, **8**, 8–14.

Sandberg, D. H., McIntosh, R. M., Bernstein, C. W., Carr, R., and Strauss, J. (1977). Severe steroid-responsive nephrosis associated with hypersensitivity. *Lancet*, **1**, 388–90.

Savilahti, E. (1981). Cow's milk allergy. *Allergy*, **36**, 73–88.

Sheffer, A. L., and Austen, K. F. (1980). Exercise-induced anaphylaxis. *J. Allergy Clin. Immunol.*, **66**, 106–11.

Soothill, J. F. (1976). Some intrinsic and extrinsic factors predisposing to allergy. *Proc. R. Soc. Med.*, **67**, 439–42.

Soter, N. A., and Austen, K. F. (1976). The diversity of mast-cell derived mediators: implications for acute, subacute and chronic cutaneous inflammatory disorders. *J. Invest. Dermatol.*, **67**, 313–19.

Speer, F. (1973). Management of food allergy. In: *Immunology in Children* (eds F. Speer and R. J. Dockhorn). C. C. Thomas, Springfield, Illinois, pp.397–402.

Speer, F., Denison, T. R., and Baptist, J. E. (1981). Aspirin Allergy. Ann. Allergy **46**, 123–6.

Squire, J. R. (1952). Tissue reactions to protein sensitization. *Br. Med. J.*, **1**, 1–7.

Stenius, B. S. M., and Lemola, M. (1976). Hypersensitivity to acetyl salicylic acid (ASA) and tartrazine in patients with asthma. *Clin. Allergy*, **6**, 119–27.

Tabuenca, J. M. (1981). Toxic–allergic syndrome caused by ingestion of rapeseed oil denatured with aniline. *Lancet*, **2**, 567–8.

Turner, M. W., Mowbray, J. F., Harvey, B. A. M., Brostoff, J., Wells, R. S., and Soothill, J. F. (1978). Defective yeast opsonization and C2 deficiency in atopic patients. *Clinc. Exp. Immunol.*, **34**, 253–9.

Unsworth, D. J., Kieffer, M., Holborrow, E. J., Coombs, R. R. A., and Walker-Smith, J. A. (1981). IgA anti-gliadin antibodies in coeliac disease. *Clin. Exp. Immunol.*, **46**, 286–93.

Vaz, G. A., Tan, L. K. T., and Gerrard, J. W. (1978). Oral cromoglycate in treatment of adverse reactions to foods. *Lancet*, **1**, 1066.

Vicario, J. L., Serrano-Rios, M., SanAndres, F., and Arnaiz-Villena, A. (1982). HLA-DR3, DR4 increase in chronic stage of Spanish oil disease. *Lancet*, **1**, 276.

Waldman, T. A., Wochner, R. D., Laster, L., and Gordon, R. S. (1967). Allergic gastroenteropathy; a cause of excessive gastrointestinal protein loss. *N. Engl. J. Med.*, **276**, 761–9.

Warin, R. P., and Smith, R. J. (1976). Challenge test battery in chronic urticaria. *Br. J. Dermatol.*, **94**, 401–6.

Wasserman, S. I., Goetzl, E. J., and Austen, K. F. (1975). Inactivation of slow reacting substance of anaphylaxis by human eosinophil arylsulphatase. *J. Immunol.*, **114**, 645–9.

Whitfield, M. F., and Barr, D. G. D. (1976). Cow's milk allergy in the syndrome of thrombocytopenia with absent radius. *Arch. Dis. Child.*, **51**, 337–43.

Wilson, J. F., Heiner, D. C., and Lahey, M. E. (1964). Milk-induced gastro-intestinal bleeding in infants with hypochronic microcytic anaemia. *J. Am. Med. Assoc.*, **189**, 568–72.

Wraith, D. G. (1980). Respiratory diseases. In: *Proceedings of the First Food Allergy Workshop* (ed. R. R. A. Coombs). Medical Education Services, Oxford, pp.64–8.

Wraith, D. G., Young, G. V. W., and Lee, T. H. (1979). The management of food allergy with diet and Nalcrom. In: *The Mast Cell: its Role in Health and Disease* (eds J. Pepys and A. M. Edwards). Pitman Medical, Tunbridge Wells, pp.443–6.

Wright, R., and Truelove, S. C. (1965). Circulating antibodies to dietary proteins in ulcerative colitis. *Br. Med. J.*, **2**, 142–4.

Zeiger, R. S., Yurdin, D. L., and Colten, H. R. (1976). Histamine metabolism. II. Cellular and subcellular localization of the catabolic enzymes, histamine methyl transferase, in human leukocytes. *J. Allergy Clin. Immunol.*, **58**, 172–9.

False Food Allergies:
Non-Specific Reactions to Foodstuffs

D. A. Moneret-Vautrin

Professeur Agrégé — Service de Médecine 'D'
(Médecine Interne et Immuno-Allergologie)
Vandoeuvre-les-Nancy, France

Those alimentary disorders which come to mind under the name of 'food allergy' have remained ill-defined and controversial because of three difficulties:

(1) confusion about the terms used and their meanings (allergy? pseudo-allergy? intolerance?);
(2) lack of knowledge of the complex defence mechanisms of the digestive tract — both immunological and non-immunological — which deal with the potentially harmful effects of foods;
(3) contradictory opinions on the reliability, sensitivity, and therefore the practical use of different diagnostic tests.

The pathological processes, and the foods which cause them, provide classical examples of toxicity, idiosyncrasy, and allergy. The apparent difference is the variable degree of responsibility attributed to the organism and the foodstuff. In toxicity everything depends on the food. In idiosyncrasy a food is responsible for a reaction in certain individuals who show an anomaly (enzymatic). In allergy, any food can bring about disorders by means of a particular immunological reaction that can be subdivided into four types, the most common of which are Type I (immediate) and Type IV (delayed).

If the physician can exclude those rare illnesses which are due to acute toxicity and the uncommon problems of chronic toxicity, he still remains confronted by intolerance or idiosyncrasy (with known, suspected, or unknown pharmacological mechanisms) and allergy (immunological mechanisms).

For a long time the confusion between intolerance and allergy has resulted from a clinical approach and a form of reasoning that can be schematized as follows: 'as there are urticarias caused by allergy to fish, then all fish-induced urticaria is due to allergy'. This is the confusion between the allergic symptom (due, in the case considered, to specific IgE) and the histamine-induced symptom. (It is true that histamine is released by the action of IgE but important to note that it is capable of being released directly without the help of antibodies.)

We have suggested the term false food allergies (FFA) to characterize the totality of illness appearing in the guise of an immediate allergy related to a non-specific histamine mechanism (Moneret-Vautrin and Grilliat, 1981). We have been led to identify the categories of foods, grouping together foods which are not chemically related but which contain a common substance, or bring about the same effects. In our view, the establishment of a FFA rests on the conjunction of three anomalies:

(1) excess consumption of one or the other of these categories of food is likely to cause a disorder, directly or indirectly, by a histamine mechanism — this alimentary disorder occurs against a particular metabolic background;
(2) the digestive mucous membrane appears functionally altered (Lessof *et al.*, 1980), which leads to an abnormal passage of foodstuffs into the circulation, both in quantity and timing;
(3) the organism has an abnormal tendency to release histamine or is hyper-reactive to histamine.

Thus defined, FFA consist of illnesses caused by histamine-releasing foods, reactions to foods which are rich in histamine, intolerance to tyramine and phenyl-ethylamine, intolerance to sodium nitrite, and histamine-induced illnesses provoked by starchy foods and alcohols. This framework is likely to accommodate many types of food intolerance which present with the same symptoms, even where it is subsequently shown that the causative agent is not solely histamine and where prostaglandins and leukotrienes may be involved (Buisseret, 1980; Debry, 1980; Doeglas *et al.*, 1967; Freedman, 1977a,b; Gallagher *et al.*, 1978; Gerber *et al.*, 1979; Harada *et al.*, 1981; Heim and Froese, 1981; Henderson and Raskin, 1972; Juhlin, 1981; Juhlin *et al.*, 1972; Kaufmann *et al.*, 1977; Kubberor *et al.*, 1974; Kushe, 1975; Lessof *et al.*, 1979). This extensive group of disorders includes adverse reactions to food additives.

A good number of previous observations, published in the United States, concern subjects who are said to be allergic to cheeses, red wines, chocolate, cereals, etc. These 'alimentary polysensitizations' have thrown discredit on the concept of food allergy but should very probably go under the heading of FFA, which appears to us to be much more frequent than food allergy itself. We shall consider successively FFA and adverse reactions to food additives.

PATHOPHYSIOLOGY OF FFA

Apart from immunological protective mechanisms, it is advisable to consider protective mechanisms against histamine (and certain amines). They are involved at two levels (Moneret-Vautrin *et al.*, 1981):

(1) *At the intestinal level:* Parrot (1949) and Mordelet-Dambrine and Parrot (1970) have shown in the guinea-pig how important are the mucoproteins which are secreted locally by the intestinal epithelium. These mucoproteins pass into the intestinal juice or cover the brush border of the enterocytes (glycocalix). Their richness in carbohydrate makes them resistant to proteolysis, and they fix and inactivate a certain amount of histamine. That part which is unfixed at this level passes into the mucosa and is subject to enzymatic destruction (monoamine oxidase and acetylase) or undergoes phagocytosis by the eosinophils (Kushe, 1975; Lindhall, 1960; Marley and Thomas, 1976).

(2) *At the hepatic level:* histamine which is transmitted through the portal vein is susceptible to degradation by histaminase (Lindhall, 1960). The synthesis of this enzyme is decreased by 50 per cent in viral hepatitis (Stopik *et al.*, 1974). In man, the instillation of histamine by duodeno-jejunal tube (a double-blind test we devised) confirms the harmlessness of large doses, in the healthy subject, in amounts up to 2.75 mg/kg. Thus a bolus of 165–200 mg of histamine in an adult of average weight who has no digestive or alimentary disorders will only cause a flushed face after an interval of some minutes, persisting for no more than 10 minutes. We carried out this study in volunteers who were undergoing surgery for gall stones, in whom cholecystectomy afforded an opportunity to take blood from the portal vein. There is no significant rise in portal vein histamine level, when estimated before and 5 minutes after the administration by duodenojejunal tube of 1.2 mg/kg of histamine (i.e. 72 mg of histamine). The rise is not great (at the limit of significance) for a bolus of from 1.8 to 2.4 mg/kg of histamine (i.e. from 108 to 144 mg of histamine) (See Tables 1 and 2). It is thus clear that in healthy subjects, absorbed histamine is unlikely to account for systemic effects. This might not apply, however, in the following circumstances: first, when histaminase levels are reduced (as they would be by isoniazid) or when diamine oxidase levels are low; second, where — as in hepatic cirrhosis — there may be substantial shunts of portal blood directly into the systemic circulation; third, when an abnormal permeability of the duodeno-jejunal mucosa leads to a sudden influx of histamine. In our experience, the third possibility is the most frequent.

It may also be necessary to consider whether histamine release could be triggered at sites which are distant from the gastrointestinal tract, or

TABLE 1   Rise in portal vein histamine level after instilling histamine dichlorhydrate (HD) into the small intestine

Group	Number of subjects	HD instilled (mg)	Portal vein histamine	Peripheral vessel histamine	Portal histamine after HD	Rise in portal vein histamine
1	10	—	82 ± 39	$80 \pm 22*$	—	
2	12	120	—	—	150 ± 89	
3	17	180–240	139 ± 60	$129 \pm 55*$	161 ± 44	$p < 0.03$
4	5	300	126 ± 34	$147 \pm 96*$	294 ± 67	$p < 0.0001$

* No significant difference from portal vein histamine.

TABLE 2   Relationship between portal venous and peripheral vessel histamine levels after small intestinal bolus of histamine (same subjects as in Table 1)

Group	Number of subjects	HD instilled (mg)	Portal histamine after HD	Peripheral vessel histamine after HD*	p
2	12	120	150 ± 89	113 ± 77 (115 ± 76)	ns
3	17	180–240	161 ± 44	150 ± 72 (129 ± 55)	ns
4	5	300	294 ± 67	129 ± 48 (130 ± 65)	<0.03

* Figures in parentheses represent peripheral vessel histamine levels before instilling histamine dichlorhydrate (HD).
ns = not significant.

alternatively, whether agents such as tyramine may have effects of the same type as those which are seen with histamine. Some of these possibilities remain to be evaluated.

CLINICAL PATTERNS OF FFA

By definition, clinical patterns mimic those of food allergy, but the symptoms are less clearly delineated. They are essentially chronic urticaria, recurrent vasomotor headaches, and intestinal functional problems (slow digestion, meteorism, abdominal pains, intermittent diarrhoea).

Histamine shock may occur but is less dramatic than anaphylactic shock and appears much later. One to three hours after the meal the subject has a feeling of warmth, with general erythema, nausea, vomiting, or diarrhoea. This can be combined with a moderate and transient fall in blood pressure. When treated with antihistamines or, in severe cases, with intramuscular cortico-steroids, the symptoms disappear within a few hours.

THE PRINCIPAL TYPES OF FFA

We shall consider successively the FFA due to non-specific histamine release, excess histamine, intolerance to tyramine and phenylethylamine, intolerance to sodium nitrite, and reactions to starchy foods and alcohol.

Illnesses due to non-specific histamine release

Since Paton (1958), who first coined the term 'histamine releasers', it has been shown that there are numerous histamine-releasing agents. Paton postulated that any molecule having at least two basic groups (amine, amidine, isothiourea, or quaternary groupings), which is separated by an aliphatic chain of five atoms of carbon or more, or by an aromatic skeleton, must be presumed to be capable of releasing histamine. This principle led to the synthesis of 48/80, a powerful histamine releaser.

Among the proteinic histamine-releasing agents, the endogenous poly-peptides of the neutrophils and eosinophils are well known, as well as the anaphylatoxins (C_{3a} and C_{5a}) generated by the activation of the alternative pathway of the complement. Among the exogenous polypeptides are the poisons of reptiles and bees (melittin) and the proteases (chymotrypsin). Included in this group are the lectins (of vegetable origin) such as concanavalin-A (Helm and Froese, 1981) and the oligopeptides, as studied in particular by Stanworth (1980).

Certain foods also possess a histamine-releasing action: egg-white—because of ovomucoid (Schachter and Talesnik, 1952)—shellfish, strawberries, tomatoes (Schachter, 1956), chocolate, fish, and pork. Similar effects are also caused by pineapple and pawpaw (containing proteolytic enzymes) and ethanol (ethyl alcohol). We can even predict the histamine-releasing effect of leguminous plants, peanuts, and cereals (Helm and Froese, 1981) by the lectins they contain.

Histamine-release illnesses follow a different course in children and in adults.

Young children

In the young child (most often between 3 and 8 years old), this type of disorder is often observed when there is an atopic background (atopic dermatitis, asthma due to dusts, or hay fever). From this fact we can be led to believe that here is a particular tendency to release histamine. The child, though not weighing a great deal, is greedy, and the ingestion of histamine-releasing foods which he likes (strawberry, chocolate) is excessive.

Apart from the common histamine-dependent symptoms (urticaria, Quincke's oedema), there may be an exacerbation of aphthous stomatitis or of atopic dermatitis, neither of which is in this case due to food allergy. It is well known that eczematous skin is very rich in mast cells. Histamine will be released there in greater quantities than elsewhere, and the pruritis will cause a scratching which accentuates the lesions. Conversely, if the histamine-releasing effect is not too pronounced the child, once cured of his eczema, will be able to ingest the food (e.g. egg-white) without causing a reaction.

The growing child becomes less sensitive to histamine release as he gets older. After 8 years of age the incriminating foodstuffs can be ingested in normal quantities without causing a reaction. The patient, however, faithfully retains the notion of the 'allergy to strawberries' that never was. More than a hundred of these subjects were studied by skin tests and human basophil degranulation tests: not one case was positive.

Adults

In the adult, non-specific histamine-release effects result from the excessive consumption of 'fast' or ready made foods (chocolate, egg, deep-frozen fish, pork chops, tomatoes, etc.). Without distinctive clinical characteristics this possibility of pseudo-allergy to food is rarely identified. This may be because there are other foods which also contribute, or because the development of urticaria is encouraged by factors such as fatigue and an anxiety state often equated in France with 'spasmophilia' and accompanied by neuromuscular hyperexcitability, which becomes manifest during hyperventilation; or in other cases because the digestive mucous membrane shows itself to be hyper-permeable. An example is provided by the individual who develops localized urticaria and erythema on the forehead (or more florid symptoms of histamine shock), in the quarter of an hour following the taking of an aperitif on an empty stomach, accompanied by the ingestion of peanuts, almonds, etc.

Illnesses due to histamine excess

The first reported cases concern cheeses and tuna fish. Doeglas and his colleagues (1967) reported the observation of a young man who developed an erythema with headaches and fall in blood pressure after eating an old cheese (Gouda), containing 85 mg of histamine per 100 g. Boyer *et al.* (1965) studied an 'epidemic' which affected 25 per cent of subjects who had eaten tuna fish containing up to 400 mg of histamine per 100 g. At present, cooked pork meats, sauerkraut, and fermented cheeses are the common causes of this syndrome. Quevauviller and N'Guyen Van Hoa (1965) have made a detailed review of the food sources of histamine (Table 3).

TABLE 3   Foods rich in histamine ($\mu g/g$)

Fermented cheeses	up to 1330
Fermented drinks (wine)	20
Fermented foods	
sauerkraut	160 mg/kg
	(a portion of 250 g = 40 mg)
Dry pork and beef sausage	225
Pig's liver	25
Tinned tuna	20
Tinned anchovy fillets	33
Tinned smoked herring's eggs	350
Tinned foods	from 10 to 350
Meats	10
Vegetables	traces
Tomato	22
Spinach	37.5
Deep-frozen fish	1
Fish, fresh shellfish	0.2
Fish:	
tuna	5.4
sardine	15.8
salmon	7.35
anchovy fillets	44

Illnesses due to intolerance to tyramine

It was in 1967 that Hanington first drew attention to the part played by tyramine in the origin of certain migraines, showing that the ingestion of 100 mg of tyramine provokes headaches which are vasomotor, temporal, and either uni- or bilateral, often with local cutaneous erythema, beginning after a delay of 2 to 15 hours. Tyramine can also provoke urticaria, and in patients who have chronic urticaria, the ingestion of 100 mg can provoke an attack in 11 per cent of cases, 40 mg being sufficient to cause a reaction in 5 per cent of cases. The mechanism is not unique. On the one hand, tyramine is a histamine releaser. On the other, during its passage in the lung, it would be expected to liberate prostaglandins and other vaso-active agents capable of acting on the cerebral vessels. The factors which provoke the symptoms of intolerance to tyramine are (Bonnet and Nepveux, 1971):

(1) excessive consumption of foods which are rich in it (Table 4);
(2) excessive endogenous synthesis by decarboxylation of tyramine caused by the intestinal flora;
(3) a partial deficiency of platelet monoamine oxidase, leading to incomplete degradation.

TABLE 4   Foods rich in tyramine* (μg/g)

French cheeses:	
Camembert	20–86
Brie	180
Gruyère	516
Cheddar	1466
Roquefort, hung game	High but variable
Brewer's yeast	1500
Soused herrings	3030
Chianti	25

Chocolate contains methyltyramine
*See also Chapter 8

Intolerance to phenylethylamine

Vasomotor headaches can follow the ingestion of chocolate. One postulated mechanism involving tyramine was refuted by Sandler *et al.* (1970) when an analysis carried out by the British Food Manufacturing Industries Research Association did not find this substance in chocolate. On the other hand, chocolate contains phenylethylamine (1 mg/15 g segment), a substance also found in numerous cheeses and red wines. The ingestion of 3 mg, in 38 subjects who had had headaches provoked by chocolate, brought about the symptoms in 16 of them after 12 hours.

Intolerance to sodium nitrite (E350)

This preservative is an excellent anti-oxidizing, anti-microbial agent (and is particularly effective against *Clostridium botulinum*). By reacting with haemoglobin and myoglobin it forms nitrite derivatives which are responsible for the 'nice pink colour' of cooked pork meats. It is still used in cheese, pickles in brine (Dutch Gouda or Edam), and various herring preparations. The maximum legal content is 15 mg/100 g of any food product in France (62 mg/100 g in the USA).

The authorized daily dose (ADD) in both France and Great Britain is 0.2 mg/kg, and this figure is widely accepted (i.e. 4 mg/day for a child of 20 kg; 12 mg/day for an adult of 60 kg). The daily consumption commonly exceeds this figure, particularly in the child.

When oral provocation tests are performed with 20 mg sodium nitrite, we have obtained positive results in 5.2 per cent of suspect cases, giving rise to attacks of urticaria, intestinal functional disorders, or vasomotor headaches, all of which appear to be attributable to this additive (Moneret-Vautrin et al., 1980). Others have noted similar side-effects; and in 1972, Henderson and Raskin published a case of vasomotor headache caused by sodium nitrite. It seems certain that symptoms which were hitherto blamed on an allergy to pork, or on an excess of histamine in cooked pork meats are frequently due to this additive.

The mechanism by which sodium nitrite acts is unclear. The denaturation of the mucoproteins by the reducing effect of sodium nitrite on —SH groups (Kubberor et al., 1974) probably leads to a 're-release' of absorbed histamine and to a disorganization of the molecular structure of secretory IgA. Sodium nitrite, by causing cellular anoxia, might also inhibit the enzymatic activity of the monoamine oxidases. Both of these effects might interfere with the protective mechanisms of the intestinal mucous membrane with regards to various antigens and chemical substances present inside the intestine (Saint-Blanquat, 1980).

Starchy foods

An excessive intake of starchy foods (which also contain cellulose) results in an increase of the processes of fermentation and an increased growth of the intestinal flora which is responsible for it. On the one hand the products (organic acids) are irritants for the colonic mucous membrane; on the other, the intestinal flora synthesizes histamine which can then pass into the circulation.

FFA due to intolerance to alcohol

The taking of alcohol in excessive quantities is noted in 38 per cent of the subjects showing a FFA. In this case the alcohol plays a stimulating role due to more than one action. By bringing about vasodilatation it facilitates the rapid passage of foods across the intestinal mucous membrane. Apart from this its aldehyde, ethanal, is a potent histamine releaser.

More rarely intolerance to wines and other alcoholic beverages is not related to a high intake but occurs as an isolated phenomenon caused by relatively small quantities. The observable symptoms are a flush, palpitations, tachycardia, muscular weakness, or respiratory symptoms, rhinitis or asthma (Breslin et al., 1973). Allergy to grapes is exceptional, as are allergies to cereals or potatoes (intolerance to whisky or vodka).

The mechanisms of intolerance are numerous:

(1) the histamine-releasing action of ethanal;
(2) the richness of histamine in certain red or white wines;
(3) intolerance to benzoates, which are contained in great quantity in certain grapes;
(4) intolerance to the quinine contained in certain aperitifs;
(5) intolerance to certain preservatives, such as sulphur dioxide.

Harada has recently shown that vasomotor and cardiac problems arise preferentially in subjects with hepatic aldehyde dehydrogenase deficiencies, in association with a raised level of blood acetaldehyde. This would be characteristic of 50 per cent of the population of Japan (Harada et al., 1981).

THE DIAGNOSIS OF FFA (Fig. 1)

In the search for an alimentary cause involving the food categories which have been described above, it is essential to analyse the dietary intake of amines and nitrites, as well as starch and dairy foods, coffee, and alcoholic beverages.

The assessment begins with the study of the patient's diet over a period of a week, in which the objective is to analyse all ingested substances in categories which include foods which are rich in tyramine or histamine or which release histamine, starchy foods, milk, and dairy products, alcohol or coffee. The subject notes down all the food and liquid which is taken, together with the quantity. This list is then analysed, both in quantity and category, assigning one point to a 'usual quantity' of each particular food. The same food may appear simultaneously in 2 or 3 different categories, and the total of weekly points for each category is reduced to an average daily index, to be compared with a normal range obtained from a group of randomly chosen healthy subjects.

Initially, this type of enquiry allowed us to establish the frequency of ingestion of food additives and to identify the provocation tests which were indicated in individual cases. We have since continued to use it clinically, and have found it valuable as a diagnostic tool.

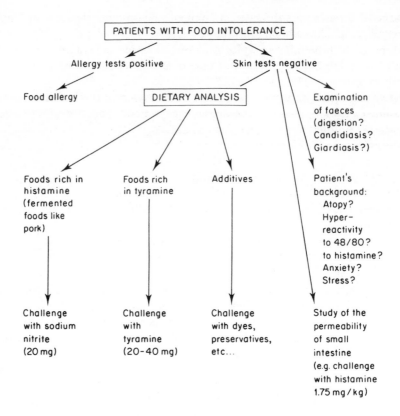

FIGURE 1   The diagnosis of false food allergy

The study of the intestinal mucous membrane

It is important to enquire about the current use of acetylsalicylic acid or non-steroidal anti-inflammatory drugs, irritant laxatives, and antibiotic treatment.

Two examinations can be useful: the examination of faeces for the level of total organic acids and fats, and a search for candidosis or giardiasis; possibly, too, the response to a duodenal bolus of histamine (1.75 mg/kg) which should normally be tolerated without any other sign but a flushed face for a few minutes. This type of challenge must, however, be performed in a double-blind study.

The metabolic response to histamine

This is estimated by non-specific histamine-release skin tests with the compound 48/80 and the reactivity to histamine. Evidence of alkalosis or latent tetany is sought by Chvostek's sign, electromyography, or by evidence of either a diminished cellular magnesium or a reduced blood level of ionized calcium or potassium.

ADVERSE REACTIONS TO ADDITIVES

Food additives are substances which are legally added to food with the aim of ensuring a precise action: preservation, colouring, etc. A number of these are also used in the pharmaceutical and cosmetics industries. The frequency of reactions to additives is different to assess. The Danish study led by Poulsen assessed it as 0.1 per cent. Juhlin was in agreement with this. The European Economic Community study group came back with a margin of between 0.03 and 0.15 per cent.

The additives are responsible for a number of clinical disorders (EEC Study, 1981). Chronic urticaria is one of the most frequent of these. When provocation tests are carried out, one or more additives have been incriminated in a third of cases, according to Juhlin: azo-dyes in 18 per cent; benzoates in 11 per cent; annatto in 10 per cent; butylhydroxyanisol (BHA) and butylhydroxytoluene (BHT) in 15 per cent; quinoline yellow in 13 per cent (Juhlin, 1981; Juhlin et al., 1972). Asthmatic reactions are also much more common than was thought and are related to the ingestion of chemical substances with low molecular weights (Freedman, 1977a).

First of all, attention has been drawn to those subjects who show an association between nasal polyposis, late-appearing non-reaginic asthma, and an intolerance to acetylsalicylic acid and to non-steroidal anti-inflammatory drugs. It has been shown that about 20 per cent of these patients have a reaction, on testing, to food additives (above all tartrazine and sodium benzoate). In an exhaustive study Schlumberger (1980) arrived at the following frequencies of reactions: anti-inflammatories and analgesics, 48 per cent; additives, 16 per cent; other substances, 36 per cent.

Anaphylactic shock has been noted after the injection of artificial colours such as patented blue V used for the location of lymphatics, or indigo blue used for the location of ureters. This hazard should be borne in mind when planning a provocation test, which aims at diagnosis, in a patient who has a history of being particularly sensitive to the tested colourant (Moneret-Vautrin and Aubert, 1978).

It has also been suggested by Feingold that the hyperactive-child syndrome (consisting of incessant agitation, inability to fix attention, and aggressiveness) may be caused by an overconsumption of colourants. The studies of Swanson and Kinsbourne (1980), using 150 mg capsules of six mixed colourants (the most common) supported this hypothesis, but the evidence for this vogue diagnosis and for its food-induced origin has been much criticized by others.

The mechanisms of adverse reactions to additives are varied. They are generally substances with low molecular weights, which are ingested irregularly in very small doses. On the evidence which is available, adverse effects due to various pharmacological mechanisms may be much more common than the effects of sensitization and the mechanisms of allergy.

Immuno-allergic responses to additives

Landsteiner's work first suggested that immunological responses can be provoked by dinitrobenzene derivatives, thanks to their ability to bond covalently with macromolecules. He therefore developed the concept of haptenes, made immunogenic by their linking to a carrier protein. Penicillin, chrome and nickel salts, textile colouring agents, certain quinones, toluene di-isocyanate (TDI), platinum salts, etc. (Pepys *et al.*, 1979) have, in turn, been shown to be capable of acting in this way, and IgE reactions have been reported to at least some of these substances.

It has been suggested that certain additives can play this role of haptenes, particularly azo-dyes. Amongst these is tartrazine. 1-sulphophenyl-3-carboxy-(4-sulphophenyl-azo)-pyrazol can combine with a protein, such as human serum albumin, by covalent bonding in the presence of a catalyst or after reacting with phosphorus pentachlorides, and it then gives rise to reactive sulphonyl groupings with the primary amine groups of proteins (Brighton, 1981). However, without a catalyst the linking constant of tartrazine with albumin serum (human or bovine) seems weak (Kauffman *et al.*, 1977). If immunological reactions are provoked by azo-dyes it is therefore possible that more reactive metabolites could be the responsible haptenes (such as sulphanilic acid and the pyrazolone derivative in the case of tartrazine) or that the reaction is directed against the impurities which are present in certain colourants (Menoret, 1979). The existence of IgE antibodies against tartrazine has nevertheless been demonstrated experimentally (Moneret-Vautrin *et al.*, 1979) and has been confirmed in man by the RAST technique for numerous colourants, including amaranth red, green S, sun yellow (Brighton, 1981). Weliky and his colleagues (1979) have also discovered IgD specific to tartrazine in six allergic subjects. The exact role of these antibodies has not been established.

After exposure to artificial colours and other types of chemical substance, a delayed type of hypersensitivity is also possible, showing itself by eczema after ingestion of an additive (azo-dyes, BHT and BHA, parabens, quinine, etc.). The mechanism is unknown, but it has been postulated that type IV sensitization develops originally after skin contact with the additive—example, after occupational contact in the food, ointments, or cosmetics industries.

Pharmacological mechanisms of the intolerance to additives

Theoretically, food additives might interfere with the synthesis of prostaglandins and leukotrienes or might activate bradykinin, potentiate the release of certain neuro-transmitters, compete with them, or inhibit their synthesis. There is some evidence to suggest that mechanisms of this kind can operate in man. Thus, asthma caused by acetylsalicylic acid or tartrazine might be the consequence of their inhibitory action on cyclo-oxygenase, provoking the inhibition of prostaglandin synthesis, particularly PGE_2 which is normally a bronchodilator (Gerber et al., 1979). Gallagher et al. (1978) claimed to show the inhibition of platelet aggregation by tartrazine, and while Vargaftig et al. (1980) could not confirm this observation in normal subjects, they suggested that there was a different susceptibility for pulmonary and platelet enzymes. A direct effect upon the synthesis of prostaglandins may not be the only mechanism involved. In fact, present knowledge of the balance of the synthesis of prostaglandins and leukotrienes (the production of which increases when the synthesis of prostaglandins is slowed down) invites us to attribute tartrazine-induced asthma to a leukotriene effect (Borgeat, 1981). Despite an extensive interest in other mediators, it may be worth noting that only one group (Neuman et al., 1978) has supported the hypothesis that the activation of bradykinin might provide an alternative explanation for these disorders due to tartrazine.

Certain colouring agents (xanthenes and erythrosin) alter the membrane permeability of neurones. Erythrosin facilitates the release of neurotransmitter at the neuromuscular junction (in a study carried out on the frog). This effect is independent of calcium and it is suggested that such an interference with neuronal conduction could be the cause of behavioural disorders seen in animals and humans, after ingesting colouring agents (Augustine and Levitan, 1980).

The search for evidence of an effect of food additives on human behaviour remains speculative. It has been suggested that monosodium glutamate would be likely to compete with gamma-aminobutyric acid, which is a neurotransmitter, and so bring about an increased production of synaptic acetylcholine, leading to neural conduction problems. There is, however, no evidence that this occurs. Finally, Stokes and Scudder (1974) have shown that butylated hydroxytoluene and hydroxyanisole caused a fall in serotonin, cholinesterase activity, and the level of cerebral noradrenaline in a newborn mouse which had been exposed in utero. Regardless of the mechanism, these additives were found to provoke behavioural disorders (aggressiveness, sleep, orientation) in these animals (Stokes et al., 1972; Stokes and Scudder, 1974).

THERAPEUTIC PROCEDURE IN FFA
AND ADVERSE REACTIONS TO ADDITIVES

The correction of dietetic errors is of the utmost importance. Since the beginning of the century food consumption in France has undergone great changes, with an increase of sugars, fruits, and vegetables, as well as cooked pork meats (which doubled between 1950 and 1968) (Meyer, 1975). Similar developments have been noted in other countries. Since 1965 the consumption of vegetables has gone down, whilst there has been an increase (in 1974) of 18 per cent in the consumption of eggs. There are some local differences in eastern France, where the consumption of meat, green vegetables, and fruits is at its lowest. We can suppose that these have been replaced by starchy and sugary foods in this part of the country. On the other hand, storage provides an added problem, and the length of time spent on the commercial circuit makes fish a cause of histamine-induced illnesses (histidine changes to histamine during storage). Thus, we can see histamine-provoked symptoms which are dependent on the changes of consumption and regional eating habits. In the child, the present excess of sugary foods, well known among nutritionists (Debry, 1982), conceals a regular consumption of additives (preservatives and colourants) which the allergist must systematically take into account. Finally, certain reducing diets (based on the intake of a single food during a week) seem to us to encourage the development of symptoms which are histamine-mediated.

At present, we do not have much evidence about average eating habits with regards to the above foods. In its absence, the rule in clinical treatment is to re-establish a balanced and varied everyday diet, free from alimentary or pharmacological irritants. It is never a question of totally eradicating a category of food, but of restricting an excessive intake. However, a diet which eliminates food additives, as proposed by Freedman (1977b), seems reasonable and worth considering in certain children. In the most severe cases, where there is a strong suggestion of food allergy but no evidence as to its cause, the institution of parenteral feeding can precede the careful resumption of oral feeding, with a progressive reintroduction of various foods.

Some general measures may be of some value:

(1) regular meal-times, which presupposes those of work and sleep;
(2) the protection of the epithelium by bland agents (colloidal aluminium phosphate and hydrochloric lemonade are popular in France, pancreatic enzymes and cellulases on occasions, and sulphurated drugs in children);
(3) protective measures directed at the mucous membrane—the possible complementary role of anti-H_2 drugs (cimetidine) must be added to the classic antihistamines which block the H_1 receptors; but drugs with a coloured coating should be avoided.

In contrast to this, sodium cromoglycate does not seem very effective in adults (contrary to its action in food allergy). It appears to be effective, however, in some histamine-releasing illnesses in children.

CONCLUSIONS

Food allergy, defined immunologically, only represents a small part of alimentary pathology: false food allergies are considerably more common. Abnormal absorption or degradation of histamine, the effect of histamine releasing agents, and intolerance to tyramine, phenylethylamine, sodium nitrite and other agents may all play a part.

The notion of an individual unbalanced diet in certain food categories seems to us to play a fundamental role, in subjects whose intestinal mucosa often seems to be made more sensitive by the frequent use of non-steroidal anti-inflammatory drugs.

The increasing importance of catering services will mean that any alimentary policy that confuses the allergic and pseudo-allergic disorders could affect a great many individuals. It seems of paramount importance that both the allergist and the nutritionist should be aware of these problems.

REFERENCES

Augustine, J. G., and Levitan, H. (1980). Neuro-transmitter release from a vertebrate neuro-muscular synapse affected by a food dye. *Science*, **207**, 1489–90.

Bonnet, G. F., and Nepveux, P. (1971). Les migraines tyraminiques. *Sem. Hôp. Paris*, **47**, 2441–5.

Borgeat, P. (1981). Leukotrienes: a major step in the understanding of immediate hypersensitivity reactions. *J. Med. Chem.*, **24**, 121–6.

Boyer, J., Depierre, F., Tissier, M., and Jacob, J. (1956). Intoxications histaminiques collectives par le Thon. *Presse Med.*, **64**, 1003–4.

Breslin, A. B. X., Hendrick, D. J., and Pepys, J. (1973). Effect of disodium cromoglycate on asthmatic reactions to alcoholic beverages. *Clin. Allergy*, **3**, 71–82.

Brighton, W. D. (1981). IgE antibodies to four food colours. Communication to *Journées Franco-Britanniques d'Asthmologie*, Montpellier, 25–26 Février.

Buisseret, P. (1980). Drug treatment of allergic gastro-enteritis. *Am. J. Clin. Nutr.*, **33**, 865–71.

Debry, G. (1980). L'alimentation des enfants français est-elle satisfaisante? *Cah. Med.*, **19**, 1117–19.

Doeglas, H., Huisman, J., and Nater, J. P. (1967). Een geval van histamine-intoxicatie door he teten van kaas. *Nederlands Tijdschr. voor geneeskundrer*, **111**, 1526–9.

EEC Study (1981). Rapport sur les réactions adverses aux additifs alimentaires. Elaboré par un groups de travail de la C.E.E.

Feingold, B. F. Food additives and child development. *Hosp. Pract.* **8**, 11–12, 1973, **21**, 17–18.

Freedman, B. J. (1977a). Asthma induced by sulphur dioxide benzoate and tartrazine contained in orange drinks. *Clin. Allergy*, **7**, 407–15.

Freedman, B. J. (1977b). A dietary free from additives in the management of allergic disease. *Clin. Allergy*, **7**, 417–21.

Gallagher, J. S., Berstein, I. L., and Splansky, G. L. (1978). Inhibition of platelet aggregation by tartrazine in normal and allergic individuals. *Am. Acad. Allergy*, 34th Meeting, Phoenix, 27–28 Feb.

Gerber, J. C., Payne, N. S., Oelz, O., Nies, A. S., and Oales, J. A. (1979). Tartrazine and the prostaglandin system. *J. Allergy Clin. Immunol.*, **63**, 289–94.

Hanington, E. (1967). Preliminary report on Tyramine headache. *British Medical Journal*, **1**, 550–551.

Harada, S., Agarwal, D. P., and Goedde, H. W. (1981). Aldehyde dehydrogenase deficiency as cause facial flushing reaction to alcohol (in Japanese). *Lancet*, **2**, 982.

Helm, R. M., and Froese, A. (1981). Binding of the receptors for IgE by various lectins. *Int. Arch. Allergy Appl. Immunol.*, **65**, 81–4.

Henderson, W. R., and Raskin, N. H. (1972). 'Hot-dog' headache: individual susceptibility to nitrite. *Lancet*, **2**, 1162–3.

Juhlin, L. (1981). Recurrent urticaria: findings in 330 cases seen from 1974 to 1978. *Br. J. Dermatol.*, **104**, 369–81.

Juhlin, L., Michaëlsson, G., and Zetterstrom, O. (1972). Urticaria and asthma induced by food and drug additives in patients with aspirin sensitivity. *J. Allerg. Clin. Immunol.*, **50**, 92–8.

Kauffman, P. E., Johnson, H. M., and Peeler, J. T. (1977). Protein binding of tartrazine and aspirin: an equilibrium dialysis study. *IRCS Med. Sci.*, **5**, 175.

Kubberor, G., Cassens, R. G., and Greaser, M. L. (1974). Reaction of nitrite with sulfhydryl groups of myosin. *J. Food Sci.*, **39**, 1228–30.

Kushe, J. (1975). Oxidative deamination of biogenic amines by intestinal amine-oxydases: histamine is specially inactivated by diamine oxydase. *Physiol. Chem. Phys.*, **356**, 1485–6.

Lessof, M. H., Buisseret, P. D., Merrett, T. G., Merrett, J., Wraith, D. G., and Youlten, L. J. F. (1979). Mechanisms involving prostaglandins in food intolerance. In: *The Mast Cell—its role in health and disease.* (ed. J. Pepys and A. M. Edwards) (International Symposium, Davos, Switzerland), pp.407–10.

Lessof, M. H., Baker, R. W. R., Ferrett, J., and Jackson, P. G. (1980). Intestinal permeability in food tolerance. *Allerg. Immunopathol.*, **8**, 463.

Lindhall, K. M. (1960). The histamine methylating enzyme system in liver. *Acta Physiol. Scand.*, **49**, 114–18.

Marley, E., and Thomas, D. V. (1976). Histamine and its metabolites in cat portal venous blood and intestine after duodenal instillation of histamine. *J. Physiol.*, **263**, 273–4.

Menoret, Y. (1979). Note sur l'allergie à la tartrazine. *EEC 'Industries Colours' Group*, 7 Dec.

Meyer, F. (1975). Evolution de l'alimentation des français, 1781–1972. *Gastro-Enterol. Clin. Biol.*, **1**, 1043–51.

Moneret-Vautrin, D. A., and Aubert, E. (1978). *Le risque de sensibilisation aux colorants alimentaires et pharmaceutiques.* Masson, Paris.

Moneret-Vautrin, D. A., Demange, G., Selve, C., Grilliat, J. P., and Savinet, H. (1979). Induction d'une hypersensibilité réaginique à la Tartrazine chez le lapin Immunisation par voie digestive par le conjugué covalent Tartrazine-Séralbumine humaine. *Ann. Immunol. Inst. Pasteur*, **130C**, 419–30.

Moneret-Vautrin, D. A., Einhorn, C., and Tisserand, J. (1980). Le rôle du Nitrite de sodium dans les urticaires histaminiques d'origine alimentaire. *Ann. Nutr. Alim.*, **34**, 1125–32.

Moneret-Vautrin, D. A., Viniaker, J., Boissel, P., Noel, M., and Kim, K. (1981). Effets de l'instillation d'histamine dans l'intestin grêle chez l'homme. I. Variations de l'histaminémie portale et périphérique. *Ann. Gastro-Entérol. Hépatol.*, **17**, 395–400.

Moneret-Vautrin, D. A., and Grilliat, J. P. (1981). Allergie alimentaire, pseudo-allergie alimentaire et nutrition. *EMC 'Nutrition'*, **10386A**, 10, 9.

Mordelet-Dambrine, M., and Parrot, J. L. (1970). Action de l'histamine introduite par voie buccale ou formée dans le tube digestif. *Med. Nutr.*, **6**, 59–73.

Neuman, I., Elian, R., Nahum, H., Shaked, P., and Creter, D. (1978). The danger of yellow dyes (tartrazine) to allergic subjects. *Clin. Allergy*, **8**, 65–8.

Parrot, J. L. (1949). L'histaminémie du Cobaye après ingestion d'histamine. *J. Physiol.*, **41**, 251A–254A.

Paton, W. D. M. (1958). The release of histamine. *Prog. Allergy*, **5**, 70–138.

Pepys, J., Parish, W. E., Cromwell, O., and Hughes, E. G. (1979). Passive transfer in man and the monkey of type I allergy due to heat labile and heat stable antibody to complex salts of platinum. *Clin. Allergy*, **9**, 99–108.

Poulsen, E. (1980). Danish report on allergy and intolerance to food ingredients and food additives. At Toxicology Forum, Aspen, Colorado.

Quevauviller, A., and N'Guyen Van Hoa (1965). L'histamine dans quelques produits alimentaires d'origine occidentale ou extrême-orientale. *Bull. Soc. Scient. Hyg. Alim.*, **53**, 284–94.

Saint-Blanquat, De G. (1980). Aspects toxicologiques et nutritionnels des nitrates et des nitrites. Communication au Colloque: 'Nitrates, Nitrites et Composés N-Nitrosés dans l'alimentation de l'Homme', Dijon, 6–7 May.

Sandler, M., Youdim, M. B. H., and Hanington, E. (1970). A clinical and biochemical correlation between tyramine and migraine. *Headache*, **10–12**, 43–51.

Schachter, M., and Talesnik, J. (1952). The release of histamine by egg-white in non-sensitized animal. *J. Phys.*, **118**, 258–63.

Schachter, M. (1956). Histamine-release and the angio-oedema type of reaction. *Histamine Ciba-Found-Symp.* Churchill, London, pp.167–9.

Schlumberger, H. D. (1980). Drug induced pseudo-allergic syndrome as exemplified by acetyl-salicylic acid intolerance. In: *Pseudo-Anaphylactoid Reactions*. Karger, Basel, pp.125–203.

Stanworth, D. R. (1980). Oligopeptide-induced release of histamine. In: *Pseudo-Anaphylactoid Reactions*. Karger, Basel, pp.56–107.

Stokes, J. D., Scudder, C. L., and Karczmar, A. G. (1972). Effects of chronic treatment with established food preservatives on brain chemistry and behavior of mice. *Fed. Proc.*, **31**, 596.

Stokes, J. D., and Scudder, C. L. (1974). The effect of butylated hydroxyanisole and butylated hydroxytoluene on behavior development of mice. *Dev. Psychobiol.*, **7**, 343–50.

Stopik, D., Beger, H. G., and Bittner, R. (1974). Uber den Einfuss der Leber auf die prä- und posthepathischen Konzentrationen des Plasmahistamins beim Menschen, *Klin. Wochenschr.*, **52**, 696–8.

Swanson, J. M., and Kinsbourne, M. (1980). Food dyes impair performance of hyper-reactive children on a laboratory learning test. *Science*, **207**, 1485–6.

Vargaftig, B. B., Bessot, J. C., and Pauli, G. (1980). Is tartrazine induced asthma to inhibition of prostaglandin biosynthesis?, *Respiration*, **39**, 276–82.

Weliky, N., Heiner, D. C., Tamura, H., and Anderson, S. (1979). Correlation of tartrazine hypersensitivity with specific serum IgD levels. *Immunol. Communications*, **8**, 65–71.

Clinical Reactions to Food
Edited by M. H. Lessof
© 1983 Edda Hanington. Published by John Wiley & Sons Ltd.

Migraine

Edda Hanington

Honorary Consultant,
Princess Margaret Migraine Clinic,
Charing Cross Hospital, London.

City of London Migraine Clinic

DEFINITION OF MIGRAINE

Migraine is a headache that recurs at intervals. The pain is often felt more on one side of the head than the other and, in common migraine, is frequently associated with nausea and sometimes vomiting. In classical migraine, which is roughly half as common, these symptoms are preceded or accompanied by transient focal neurological phenomena which are usually visual but can also consist of sensory and speech disturbances.

INCIDENCE

The incidence of migraine in the general population is approximately 8 per cent. It is rare in early childhood but by the age of 11 years the incidence in both boys and girls is around 5 per cent. It rises sharply in women during the child-bearing years, reaching a peak of about 20 per cent between the ages of 20 and 45 years.

Migraine has a strong familial incidence. When I asked 500 migraine sufferers whether any members of their immediate family also suffered from migraine the following information was obtained (Hanington, 1970):

Migraine in any	Parents Grandparents Brothers Sisters	66%
	Mother	38%
	Father	14%

155

PRECIPITANTS

Stress is the most common precipitant of migraine attacks. In this context the term stress includes such states as fatigue, excitement, and anger. Hormonal factors can influence the recurrence of migraine attacks which probably accounts for the peak in women during the child-bearing years.

Hypoglycaemia and dietary factors can also precipitate attacks. It is with the latter that this chapter is concerned. However, it is important to bear in mind that the precipitants of migraine can be cumulative in effect and that, as will be described later, all the precipitants of migraine lead to an attack through a final common pathway.

DIETARY FACTORS

More than 2000 years ago Hippocrates suggested that there might be a link between the eating of certain foods and headache. We read in the Hippocratic writings that 'milk is not recommended for those who suffer from headaches' and that 'sweet wine is less likely to produce headache than is heavy wine'.

In the eighteenth century a quaker physician, John Fothergill, who was born in 1712, wrote a classic treatise on migraine and food in which he stated:

> There are some things which, in very small quantities, seldom fail to produce the sick headache in some constitutions. Such are a larger proportion than usual of melted butter, fat meats, and spices, especially common black pepper. Meat pies often contain all these things united, and are as fertile a cause of this complaint as any thing I know; so are rich baked puddings, and every thing of a similar nature. A little error in these things will seldom fail to be attended with much suffering, in many constitutions (Fothergill, 1784).

When the subject of headaches and food is discussed we would do well to heed the wise words of Edward Liveing. He spent a lifetime studying the subject of headache and published an authoritative work *On Megrim, Sick-Headache and Some Allied Disorders* in 1873. He commented:

> One way in which traditional error in such matters is propagated is I am convinced, in many cases, by our faulty methods of interrogation. On the one hand, we are too apt to accept in the hurry of routine the inferences of patients for statements of fact; and on the other, we often wring from them conformity to our views by pressing them with leading questions or anticipating what they have to say.

During the first half of the twentieth century a large number of papers were written by authors who reported links between migraine attacks and the eating of certain foods (Balyeat and Rinkel, 1931; Kallos and Kallos-Deffner, 1955; Maxwell, 1965; Walker, 1963; Unger and Unger, 1952). These authors invariably concluded that migraine is an allergic disorder and several described the success achieved by elimination diets in treating migraine sufferers (Colldahl, 1965).

The foods most commonly implicated by these investigators were milk and dairy products, including cheese. Fish, alcohol, and chocolate were also mentioned. Table 1 shows the foods cited by some of these authors.

TABLE 1   Foods which are capable of provoking migraine

Reference	Alcohol	Dairy products including cheese	Chocolate	Fish	Eggs, nuts, beans
Balyeat and Rinkel (1931)		+		+	+
Kallos and Kallos-Deffner (1955)			+	+	
Maxwell (1965)			+		
Walker (1963)		+	+	+	
Unger and Unger (1952)	+	+	+	+	+

My own interest in diet and migraine began in 1966 when I read reports about the occurrence of headache reactions in patients who were taking monoamine oxidase inhibitor (MAOI) drugs (Blackwell, 1963; Blackwell and Marley, 1964, 1966). These drugs were originally introduced into clinical practice for the treatment of tuberculosis. When an elevation of mood was noticed in some of the patients treated in this way the use of MAOIs was extended to the treatment of non-endogenous depression. In spite of the fact that thousands of patients in the USA were treated with them, no adverse reactions were reported during the first 3 years of their use. Then reports slowly accumulated of cases of severe headaches associated with a rise in blood pressure in patients receiving this treatment. Gradually it was established that the headache and pressor reactions occurred in these patients on the MAOI drugs when they ate certain foods, and in particular, cheese. Cheese was found to contain the pressor amine tyramine, the name being derived from the Greek word for cheese, turos.

In 1965 Blackwell and Mabbit, who investigated these pressor reactions, analysed a number of cheeses for their tyramine content. They found that this is related to the maturation time of the cheese, the bacterial flora, and details of manufacture. It is not related to the appearance or flavour of the cheese. They found that individual samples of a given cheese differ in tyramine content from 72 to 953 μg tyramine per gram of cheese. They also stated that in some patients on MAOI therapy as little as 6 mg of tyramine orally can provoke a hypertensive crisis. Severe headache without hypertension was also reported in some of these patients (Bethune et al., 1963).

Blackwell et al. (1967) carried out an investigation to define the characteristics of the MAOI reaction and reported the following:

> Of 25 patients on monoamine oxidase inhibitors who had a hypertensive crisis, 23 had their dietary history taken: 17 had eaten cooked or raw cheese, 2 'Marmite' (yeast extract), 1 'Marmite' and cheese, 1 pickled herring, 1 tinned milk and 1 'Complan' (a milk-based food extract).

They also reported on pressor substances present in certain foods:

Cheese:	Tyramine is the main pressor substance—up to 1.42 mg/g.
Yeast extracts:	'Marmite' and some samples of 'Bovril' (to which Marmite is added) contain tyramine and histamine (the latter may contribute to the headache) 1.0–1.6 mg of tyramine/g.
Broad beans:	Hypertension due to the amino acid 'dopa' in bean skins being converted to dopamine.
Alcohol:	Wine may contain up to 25 μg of tyramine/ml.
Fish, meat:	Contains 3.03 mg of tyramine/g (pickled herring).
Chocolate:	Contains a catechol derivative vanillin, formed during the fermentation of cocoa beans.
Complan:	This (and also milk and cream) has a high amino acid content from which amines may be formed by intestinal decarboxylating bacteria.

Blackwell et al. (1967) also explored the various factors which were operative in these reactions, namely individual variables, variables in treatment, and variables in dietary factors.

The tyramine content of various cheese and alcoholic beverages has been reported in micrograms per gram by other investigators, including Howitz et al., 1964; Udenfried et al., 1959; Sen, 1969) and Table 2 gives their findings.

When I read the reports of the headache reactions in the patients on MAOIs it occurred to me that the foods implicated in these reactions were similar to those that had been mentioned, over the years, in the literature on migraine (Hanington, 1967). The similarity is seen in Table 3. In order to obtain more precise information about dietary factors and migraine, the help of the British Migraine Association was obtained. I selected 500 migraine sufferers who

TABLE 2   Amount of tyramine in various foods ($\mu g/g$)

Cheeses		Alcoholic beverages		Other foods	
Camembert	86	Beer, Brand A	1.8	Banana pulp	7
Stilton	466	Beer, Brand B	2.3	Red plum	6
Brie	180	Beer, Brand C	4.4	Tomato	4
Emmentaler	225	Sherry	3.6	Avocado	23
N.Y. State Cheddar	1416	Sauterne	0.4	Potato	1
Processed American	50	Riesling	0.6	Spinach	1
		Chianti	25.4	Orange pulp	10
				Egg plant	3

TABLE 3   Comparison of foods linked with migraine attacks and with reactions to MAOIs

Food	Reported to precipitate attacks of migraine	Reported to precipitate headache and pressor reactions in patients on MAOI drugs
Alcohol	+	+
Cheese	+	+
Fish	+	+
Beans	+	+
Dairy produce	+	+
Chocolate	+	+
Eggs	+	
Wheat	+	
Nuts	+	
Tomatoes and other foods, e.g. onions, pork	+	

thought that their attacks were sometimes linked with the eating of certain foods and asked which foods they avoided eating for this reason. In order of frequency, the foods which these 500 dietary migraine sufferers cited were:

Chocolate	75%
Cheese and dairy products	48%
Citrus fruits	30%
Alcoholic drinks	25%
Fatty fried food	18%
Vegetables (especially onions)	18%
Tea and coffee	14%
Meat (especially pork)	14%
Sea food	10%

It therefore seemed worth testing whether oral tyramine could precipitate migraine in some of these sufferers, if it was given in a dose similar to that contained in 4 oz (113 g) of a cheese rich in tyramine. Patients with hypertension and those on MAOIs, were excluded from the investigation.

In a trial of this nature a patient with very frequent headaches — say, two or three a week — is obviously unsuitable. The ideal choice is someone whose attacks occur every 10–14 days, thus allowing the test substance to be given 5 or 6 days after the last headache ended, and 5 or 6 days before the next attack is expected.

Another attack of migraine is unlikely within 3 days of a previous one, so it is useless to test a patient less than 3 days after the end of an attack. Similarly, in patients whose headaches have a regular pattern of timing, no testing should be carried out within 3 days of the expected onset of an attack. For a valid test, subjects should be approached in such a way that they do not expect to develop a headache.

To tell volunteers, as Ryan (1974) did, that they are going to be given two samples, one or both of which might precipitate a headache, introduces a large psychological factor. If patients are told that it is very hard to identify migraine precipitants in food, and that repeated sampling of substances may be necessary, then psychological factors are less likely to arise. I emphasized to all my patients that one headache on a placebo sample means getting at least seven or eight negative results on placebo testing in order to balance the unexpected result. All samples were sent by post so that personal factors could not influence the results. The reports which the patients completed 24 hours after taking the test substance were also returned by post. They were asked to take the capsules with a slice of bread and butter, since this may facilitate amine absorption.

It soon became apparent that oral tyramine could precipitate typical attacks of migraine in selected sufferers (Table 4). When the headache symptoms precipitated by oral tyramine were analysed it was clear that they showed the typical features of migraine attacks. The breakdown of these symptoms is seen

TABLE 4   Results of administration of tyramine and lactose in 50 dietary migraine patients (all patients tested at least once with tyramine and hydrochloride and lactose)

125 mg	No effect	Migraine attack
Lactose	60	6
Tyramine	20	80*

* $\chi^2 = 80.2; P < 0.001$

in Table 5 (Hanington *et al.*, 1970). The highest proportion of headaches occurred within 3 hours of taking tyramine as is seen in Table 6.

The precipitants of migraine are cumulative in effect. It is therefore not surprising that on isolated occasions as little as 25 mg of oral tyramine has been found to precipitate an attack.

TABLE 5

Symptoms	Incidence (%)
Severe headache	32
Moderate headache	28
Mild headache	40
Unilateral headache	50
Bilateral headache	40
Site unspecified	10
Fortification spectra	14
Other eye signs	62
Nausea	56
Vomiting	22

TABLE 6

Time interval in hours after taking tyramine	Percentage onset headache
0–3	36
3–6	15
6–9	0
9–12	20
12–15	20
15–18	3
18–21	3
21–24	3

Effect of tyramine on unselected population

In order to find out whether or not oral tyramine had any effect on the normally headache-free population, a study was carried out with the help of 200 volunteers (Hanington *et al.*, 1970).

Volunteers, mainly women, were enlisted from those working in hospitals. All those who were pregnant, had a blood pressure greater than 140/90, or were currently taking MAOI drugs, were excluded. Of the remaining 200, 27 gave a personal history, and of the remainder nearly 20 per cent gave a family history of migraine—suggesting a bias in selection related to an interest in migraine. The volunteers were classified into three groups: migraine (27); non-migrainous headache (69); and headache-free (104).

A double-blind design was used. Identical-looking gelatin capsules were prepared containing either tyramine (125 mg) or lactose (125 mg). Each capsule was taken between 4 and 6 p.m. After 24 hours a questionnaire was completed and when this was returned a second capsule was sent with instructions to follow the same procedure. The questionnaire covered the history of headaches or migraine, the family history of migraine, and any current medication. In addition, a full description was obtained of any headache or other symptoms experienced within 24 hours following the ingestion of the capsules.

The results are summarized in Table 7. In the 'migraine' group, six out of 27 developed an attack of migraine after tyramine. Only two of these had a clear-cut dietary history. The figure for the incidence of dietary migraine is usually considered to be less than 5 per cent, but clearly it may be higher. The type of headache in this group was similar to that found in the dietary migraine group. In the non-migrainous group the headaches precipitated by tyramine were moderate or mild, and eye symptoms and nausea were less frequent than in the migraine group. In the headache-free group the headaches precipitated by tyramine were mild. Thus tyramine appears to precipitate a spectrum of headache, ranging from severe and frequent headache in migraine subjects at one end, to mild and infrequent in headache-free subjects at the other.

TABLE 7   The effect of tyramine and lactose in 200 control subjects

	Migraine subjects*	Headache subjects*	Headache-free subjects	Total
Headache after tyramine only	6	9	3	18
Headache after lactose only	1	4	2	7
Headache after both	0	2	2	4
No effect from either	20	54	97	171
TOTALS	27	69	104	200

* Taken as a single group, migraine and headache subjects had significantly more headaches after tyramine (but not after lactose) than headache-free subjects. $\chi^2 = 10.0$, 2 DF; p / 0.01.

In carrying out these tyramine tests, capsules containing 125 mg of tyramine hydrochloride were used. Ghose *et al.* (1977) studied the response of 31 migraine sufferers to intravenous tyramine. They found that whether or not these sufferers related some of their attacks to the eating of certain foods, the migraine subjects required significantly less tyramine to increase their systolic blood pressure by 30 mmHg when compared with matched controls; 46 per cent of these migraine subjects developed headaches after the tyramine injection. None of the control subjects complained of headache.

While tyramine is the vasoactive amine that has been most thoroughly investigated in migraine, it is not the only amine concerned in dietary migraine. Cheese and alcoholic beverages, for example, contain not only tyramine but also significant amounts of betaphenylethylamine and histamine. Citrus fruits contain octopamine and synephrine. All the vasoactive monoamines concerned in migraine act both directly on blood vessels and indirectly through the liberation of adrenaline and noradrenaline from nerve endings (Hanington and Harper, 1968).

Tyramine is also found in plants, as are many other free amines formed by decarboxylation of protein and non-protein amino acids. Evans *et al.* (1979) isolated *N*-methyltyramine from the seeds of *Acacia schweinfurthii* and noted the effect of both the natural and synthetic compounds in inducing migraine. This *N*-substituted amine gave pharmacological actions identical to tyramine itself.

These findings suggested to Evans *et al.* (1979) that a food containing any amine or mixture of amines which is capable of increasing the level of noradrenaline in the susceptible subject is likely to cause migraine. They endorsed what has already been observed clinically on many occasion and concluded that the vasoactive amines present in food, which act both directly and indirectly through the liberation of noradrenaline, can have a cumulative effect.

Metabolism of tyramine (see Figure 1)

The fact that oral tyramine can precipitate typical attacks of migraine in selected sufferers led to a number of biochemical investigations. These were aimed at determining whether or not the metbolism of tyramine differs from normal in migraine subjects. The excretion of both free and conjugated forms should be considered when drawing conclusions as to the normality of excretion levels of any compound and its metabolites.

Tyramine, together with other phenolic amines, is metabolized along two main routes (Figure 1). These are sulphate conjugation of the aromatic hydroxyl group and oxidative deamination of the side-chain. It is important to bear in mind that tyramine metabolites are constantly being excreted from the body as they are derived from the decarboxylation of tyrosine residues. Studies of tyramine metabolism both before and after an oral tyramine load, in a group of migraine sufferers and control subjects, indicated that the migraine subjects excreted significantly less free tyramine as well as less conjugated tyramine at all times (Smith *et al.*, 1970). Littlewood *et al.* (1982) have shown that patients with dietary migraine have significantly lower levels of platelet phenosulphotransferase activity than either migrainous patients without a history of dietary provocation or normal controls. Of the two known human variants of this enzyme, the phenol inactivating P form was more severely involved than the M enzyme. The latter inactivates monoamines including tyramine.

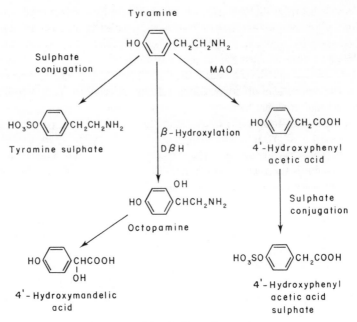

FIGURE 1   Metabolism of tyramine

Tyramine acts both directly as a sympathomimetic amine and indirectly through the release of noradrenaline. A significant increase in the excretion of catecholamines in the urine has been detected in migraine sufferers during the 3 hours after tyramine ingestion (Sandler *et al.*, 1970). Sever (1979) has suggested that the time-lapse in the development of headache following oral tyramine (Table 6) could be explained by a defect in the metabolic pathway for tyramine resulting in the formation of octopamine. This has a longer tissue half-life than tyramine, and depletes tissue catecholamines.

MONOAMINE OXIDASE

Vasoactive monoamines such as tyramine, adrenaline, betaphenylethylamine, noradrenaline, dopamine, and 5-hydroxytryptamine (5 HT) are broken down by the monoamine group of enzymes (MAO).

The MAO enzymes add oxygen and remove ammonia from amines according to the general formula:

$$RCH_2NH_2 + O_2 + H_2O \longrightarrow RCHO + NH_3 + H_2O_2$$

This enzyme is widely distributed and found in high concentrations in the liver, salivary glands, gut, kidney, stomach, and placenta (Thompson and Tickner, 1949, 1951; Southgate *et al.*, 1968).

MAO enzymes are present in the body in at least two forms: type A and type B. Work on MAO levels in migraine has been confined to platelet studies. Platelets contain MAO B. Type A is specific for 5HT and noradrenaline while phenylethylamine is the preferred substrate for type B. Tyramine and dopamine are substrates for both A and B forms. In 1970 and 1974 Sandler *et al.* reported a decrease in platelet MAO in migraine sufferers during and outside attacks. Further studies by Glover *et al.* in 1977 confirmed a significant fall in platelet MAO during migraine attacks.

The second main route by which some of the phenolic amines concerned in dietary migraine are dealt with is by the formation of sulphate conjugates. Sulphate conjugation takes place largely in the gut wall. There is some evidence of impaired sulphation at all times in migraine subjects (Smith *et al.*, 1970).

INTESTINAL FACTORS

Migraine suffers occasionally complain of the fact that their attacks have become more severe and frequent during a time when they have been taking antibiotic therapy. The use of antibiotics affects intestinal flora and this could result in increased putrefaction or decarboxylation with an increased absorption of vasoactive amines through the intestinal wall.

In a paper on pressor substances present in various foods Blackwell *et al.* (1967) mentioned milk and cream, stating that these have a high amino acid content from which amines may be formed by intestinal decarboxylating bacteria.

The high content of bacterial flora in foods such as yoghurt may also influence the breakdown of dietary amines and their absorption.

Bonnet and Nepveux (1971) carried out studies with oral tyramine in 213 migraine patients. They reported a 30 per cent incidence of headache within 18 hours of tyramine ingestion. They extended their studies to cover intestinal absorption and found that in those of their patients who developed a headache after tyramine, intestinal absorption was slower and decarboxylation processes occurred.

CHOCOLATE AND BETAPHENYLETHYLAMINE

Chocolate heads the list of foods that some migraine sufferers consider can precipitate some of their attacks. After the investigations with tyramine it was at first thought that chocolate would be found to contain this amine. This, however, was not the case. Chocolate was found to contain little or no tyramine as such. A detailed analysis of chocolate was therefore undertaken. This work was carried out, with support from the Wellcome Trust, at the British Food Manufacturers Industrial Research Association at Leatherhead under Dr M. Saxby.

Six reliable migraine patients who had previously co-operated in tyramine trials, and who all suspected chocolate of giving them a headache, agreed to test chocolate samples. These six subjects all developed typical migraine headaches within 24 hours of eating 2 oz (56 g) samples of bitter chocolate. When given samples which looked and tasted the same, but from which the amines had been removed, no headaches resulted. When the amines present in 2 oz (56 g) of chocolate were restored to test samples, headaches were again reported. The search for a possible headache precipitating factor or factors in chocolate was therefore concentrated on the identification of the amines present.

The detection of betaphenylethylamine (BPEA) aroused immediate interest as it is a vasoactive amine which acts in a similar way to tyramine on vascular tissue. Bitter chocolate is a potent headache precipitant in some dietary migraine sufferers, and samples of various brands of bitter chocolate were found to contain between 50 and 200 parts per million of BPEA. If we take the lower figure of 50 p.p.m. this means that 2 oz (56 g) of chocolate might contain up to 3 mg of BPEA. An investigation was therefore undertaken to see whether or not this amount of oral BPEA can precipitate headaches in selected migraine sufferers.

More than 60 migraine sufferers volunteered to take part in this investigation, but subjects who were known to be hypertensive or under treatment with antidepressants were excluded. All the participants completed a detailed questionnaire and were asked to obtain the consent of their own doctors before joining in the investigation. Thirty-nine people finally took part. Those taking part in the investigation were not asked to change their usual routine in any way. The method employed was the same as that originally used in the tyramine studies, and the results showed that BPEA is another amine present in food that can precipitate headaches in selected migraine subjects.

The results of this investigation showed that 3 mg of BPEA can precipitate headaches in selected migraine sufferers (Table 8). The fact that BPEA could precipitate attacks of migraine in chocolate-sensitive sufferers was important not only because of its possible role in chocolate—which contains very small amounts—but because it demonstrated that not only tyramine but also other vasoactive amines present in food can precipitate attacks.

It is extremely difficult to determine the precise amine content of chocolate, as is clear from the wide divergence in the figures reported.

Saxby analysed the BPEA content of a number of samples of cheeses, chocolates, and cocoa beans. The results are shown in Table 9. Other workers have reported much smaller amounts of BPEA in chocolate (Schweitzer et al., 1975). BPEA appears to be present in significant amounts in foods that have been fermented.

The chief headache-producing amine in chocolate may not be BPEA. Although it has not yet been positively identified it is likely that it may prove to

TABLE 8   Results of the administration of 3 mg of BPEA and identical-looking capsules containing lactose

Substance	No effect	Migraine attack
Lactose	33	6
Betaphenylethylamine (BPEA)	21	18*

* χ^2 = 8.6; p < 0.01. Two people included in this table suffered migraine attacks after taking both substances.

TABLE 9

Foodstuff		Concentration of BPEA (μg/g)
Manufacturer A	Bitter chocolate	12.3
Manufacturer B	Dairy milk chocolate	5.9
Manufacturer C	Plain chocolate	12.0
Manufacturer D	Cheddar cheese	12.8
Manufacturer E	Cheshire cheese	35.4
Manufacturer E	Mild Cheddar cheese	0
Manufacturer E	Double Gloucester cheese	10.2
Blue Stilton cheese		20.3
Unfermented cocoa beans		0
Fermented unroasted cocoa beans		1.9
Fermented roasted cocoa beans		13.1

be N-methyltyramine. This amine, like tyramine, increases blood pressure in the anaesthetized rat, relaxes guinea-pig ileum, and increases both the force and rate of contraction of guinea-pig right atrium by inducing the release of noradrenaline (Evans et al., 1979).

The seeds of *Acacia* species contain approximately 0.5 per cent dry weight of N-methyltyramine. Similar spots appear on the chromatogram for N-methyltyramine when the chromatograms of chocolate and acacia are compared (Evans and Bell, personal communication).

FOOD ADDITIVES

Substances are added to foods for a variety of reasons. They may provide attractive colouring, as in the case of tartrazine. They may be used to enhance the flavour of the food, as is the case with sodium glutamate, which gives a salty, meaty taste. Not only is sodium glutamate commonly contained in frozen-food products but it is also used in some pharmaceutical preparations such as oral preparations of liver and protein hydrolysates. Sodium nitrite is used as a colour fixative in meat products, like frankfurter sausages, bacon, and salami. All of these food additives have given rise to occasional headache reactions which have been reported in the literature.

Sodium nitrite

In 1972 Henderson and Raskin reported a series of experiments in a 58-year-old man who during the previous 7 years had developed bilateral bitemporal non-throbbing headaches when he ate cured meat such as frankfurter sausages. He was given odourless and tasteless solutions containing 10 mg or less of sodium nitrite to drink, or identical-looking solutions containing 10 mg of sodium bicarbonate. Headaches were provoked 8 out of 13 times after the ingestion of sodium nitrite but never after the ingestion of the control solution. Headaches were also provoked after the ingestion of solutions containing 100 mg of tyramine hydrochloride. These headaches usually arose within 45 minutes of the ingestion of the sodium nitrite, lasted up to 2 hours, and were sometimes associated with facial flushing. They were bitemporal, dull, and aching and not associated with visual symptoms or nausea or vomiting. In 10 volunteers with no history of food-induced headache neither sodium bicarbonate, nor sodium nitrite, nor tyramine hydrochloride provoked headaches.

Sodium glutamate

Sodium glutamate is the agent responsible for symptoms described as the 'Chinese restaurant syndrome'. The symptoms of the Chinese restaurant syndrome may arise about 15–25 minutes after a meal containing the food preservative sodium glutamate. They consist of a burning sensation in the back of the neck, across the chest, and over the forearms, together with a tightness across the chest. Approximately 5 g of sodium glutamate can produce this effect. The Chinese restaurant syndrome was first described by Schaumberg *et al.*, in 1969.

Tartrazine is an orangey-yellow powder which makes a golden yellow solution. It is a useful colouring agent for medicines and is sometimes used as a dye in foods. As little as 1 or 2 mg can sometimes give rise to asthma, urticaria, and occasionally headache in susceptible individuals.

Ice cream headache

The effect of extreme cold on nervous reflexes may account for the headache which sometimes occurs when very cold foods touch the palate. This type of headache has been termed 'ice cream headache' (Raskin and Knittle, 1976).

HISTAMINE AND HISTIDINE

Vasodilator substances and cluster headaches

Histamine is a powerful vasodilator and its possible role in vascular headache has often been considered. When 0.1 mg of histamine is given intravenously it produces flushing of the face and throbbing headache even in subjects who are normally headache-free. There is one type of headache in which histamine plays an undoubted role. This is cluster headache.

Cluster headache is thought to be a variant of migraine. As its name suggests the pain occurs in bouts or clusters. It affects men more often than women and usually begins in adult life between the ages of 30 and 40 years. The pain is extremely severe and throbbing in character. It is felt more on one side of the head than the other, usually around one eye but occasionally in the cheek or jaw. The pain is abrupt in onset, may last from a few minutes to an hour or two, and then fades away. It recurs at intervals from once to several times a day over a period of days or weeks. During the painful period the eye on the affected side often waters and becomes suffused and the nostril on the painful side of the face may become blocked. Little is known about the aetiology of cluster headache but it is associated with a significant rise in whole-blood histamine (Anthony and Lance, 1971). During a bout of attacks patients are very sensitive to vasodilator substances—and in this susceptible period the subcutaneous injection of 0.3–0.5 mg of histamine will induce a full-blown attack (Horton *et al.*, 1939), as will 1 mg of nitroglycerin sublingually. In some sufferers as little or less than an ounce of whisky, wine or beer can provoke attacks (Kudrow, 1980).

Histamine versus histidine

The formation of histamine in the gastrointestinal tract appears to depend on the presence of histidine in the diet. This is roughly proportional to the protein content. When Granerus (1968) undertook studies of histamine metabolism in man and fed eight subjects with large amounts of histamine, none of them developed any subjective or objective symptoms. When he gave four subjects each a total of 5 g of histidine in divided doses of 1 g, 2 g, and 2 g, an hour apart, all the subjects complained of headache about an hour after the last histidine intake. When I selected six reliable dietary migraine sufferers and gave them 50 mg of histamine dihydrochloride in a controlled trial, similar to the trials with oral tyramine, none of the migraine sufferers developed a headache. But when they were given 5 g capsules of L-histidine monochloride, four out of the six developed headaches within a few hours.

Controlled double-blind trials have been carried out in which the histamine H_2-receptor antagonist cimetidine was given alone, and in combination with the histamine H_1-receptor antagonist chlorpheniramine, to 24 patients with migraine and 20 patients with cluster headache. It was shown that these agents were ineffective in prophylaxis (Anthony *et al.*, 1978). The investigators suggested that the reason for this may lie in the fact that intracellular histamine does not act via receptors and concluded that histamine might still play a role in the pathogenesis of vascular headaches. It seems likely, in fact, that the effect of histamine in the body differs when it is given orally in the form of histamine or derived from the breakdown of oral histidine.

Sjaastad and Sjaastad (1977) consider that the role of histamine in vascular headache will only be satisfactorily established when techniques for the quantitative *in vivo* assessment of histamine release become available.

Clearly the possible role of histamine and histidine in vascular headache requires further investigation. Meanwhile it is worth noting the content of these substances in some foods and drinks.

Histamine is present in large amounts in some alcoholic drinks. White wines contain up to 10 mg per litre and in some red wines this figure rises to 20 mg per litre (Mayer *et al.*, 1971).

Certain cheeses and other foodstuffs containing proteolytic bacteria have a high histamine content.

Yeast extracts contain significant amounts of both tyramine and histamine. In certain vegetable extracts such as 'Marmite' the amount of histamine may reach nearly 3 mg/g (Blackwell *et al.*, 1969). These authors analysed the tyramine and histamine content of yeast extracts chromatographically and the results are shown in Table 10. Since 5 g of histidine can precipitate headache even in non-migrainous subjects it is also worth noting those foods with a high

TABLE 10

Proprietary yeast extracts	Tyramine HCl (mg/g)	Histamine HCl (mg/g)
Marmite 1	1.64	2.83
Marmite 2	1.44	1.95
Marmite 3	1.09	0.98
Salt-free 'Marmite'	0.19	1.66
Yex	0.51	1.34
Befit	0.42	0.27
Barmene	0.15	0.21
Yeastrel	0.10	0.26

histidine content. Tables giving the composition of foods (Paul and Southgate, 1978) show that the histidine content of different cheeses varies from 93 mg/100 g in cream cheese to 1050 mg/100 g in Parmesan. Camembert, Cheddar, processed cheese and Stilton contain approximately 600 mg/100 g. Both meat and fish protein contain considerable amounts of histidine but this is usually between 500 and 700 mg/100 g. The average portion of 4 oz (113 g) of meat or fish might therefore contain approximately 1 g of histidine. In roast venison the histidine content rises to 1290 mg/100 g and in lean pork chops to 1400 mg/100 g. One litre of whole milk contains only 123 mg of histidine. Peanuts, on the other hand, have a relatively high histidine content, approximately 680 mg/100 g.

Although the histidine content of a protein rich meal is very unlikely to reach 5 g of histidine, it is worth bearing in mind that in addition to their histamine content, 1 litre of some red wines can contain nearly 25 mg of tyramine and up to 10 mg of BPEA, while certain cheeses contain all the vasoactive amines commonly implicated in headache. The total vasoactive amine content of a meal consisting of meat or fish, cheese, and wine could well have a cumulative effect on a headache sufferer.

This may also be relevant to cluster headache, which is thought to be a variant of migraine. During a spell of attacks it would be worth noting the effect, if any, of foods containing considerable amounts of histamine, histidine, and vasoactive amines in general.

ALCOHOL

One in four dietary migraine sufferers consider that alcohol can sometimes precipitate an attack. There is also no doubt about the fact that alcohol can precipitate cluster headache during a bout of attacks.

Ethyl alcohol is a powerful vasodilator. Alcoholic beverages also contain several vasoactive amines, chief of which are tyramine, BPEA, and histamine. Heavy red wines, such as chianti, appear to have a more powerful headache-precipitating effect than lighter wines. It is also relevant that alcoholic beverages are often taken with snacks in the form of cheese and smoked fish, and that there is therefore a gradual build-up in the vasoactive amine content taken in the food and drink at the average cocktail party.

Mayer and Pause (1973) undertook an analysis of 56 Swiss red and white wines. Some red wines contained as much as 36 mg of tyramine and 3 mg of BPEA per litre. The tyramine content of some of the white wines investigated was as high as 20 mg/l, with up to 2 mg of BPEA per litre. Up to 15 mg histamine was found in a litre of some of these wines.

COFFEE

Migraine sufferers occasionally report a link between coffee drinking and the frequency and severity of their attacks (Selbach, 1973). Excessive coffee drinking can give rise to a number of other symptoms such as irritability, tremulousness, occasional muscle-twitching, and palpitations. Caffeine is present not only in coffee but also in other common drinks such as tea and coca cola. Coffee beans contain about 1–2 per cent of caffeine. Tea can contain as much as 4 per cent, and a small cup of strong tea could contain as much as 60 mg of caffeine. Instant coffee has a caffeine content of approximately 3–4 per cent. It may be noted, for comparison, that when caffeine is used medicinally it is given in doses of 100–300 mg.

Caffeine is a stimulant and is contained in a number of analgesic tablets. It is thought to enhance the action of ergotamine and is present in some preparations which are given for migraine, e.g. cafergot.

In a study of the effects of coffee on catecholamine excretion and plasma lipids, Froeberg *et al.* (1969) showed that the ingestion of 225 mg caffeine increased the excretion of adrenaline and noradrenaline in healthy persons. When coffee containing a high dose of caffeine (750 mg) was given, adrenaline and noradrenaline excretion were similarly increased and a small rise occurred in plasma lipids. The authors concluded that coffee and caffeine appear to be potent compounds increasing the activity in the sympatho-adrenomedullary system, with less pronounced but still significant effects on plasma lipid levels. These findings could be of relevance in migraine, where the onset of attacks is associated with an increase in catecholamine metabolism.

ALLERGY

The word allergy is included in the title of a large number of papers on migraine (Balyeat and Rinkel, 1931; Unger and Unger, 1952; Schwartz, 1952; Walker, 1963; Maxwell, 1965; Grant, 1979). However, the evidence which has been presented so far has not suggested that migraine is an allergic disorder. One of the chief reasons for regarding it so has been the fact that migraine sufferers often link a proportion of their attacks with the eating of certain foods—hardly adequate evidence of an allergic cause. Patients who fulfil all the criteria for true allergic disease (see Chapter 6) may nevertheless report an association between other symptoms of allergy and migraine attacks. It is also difficult, without introducing an allergic factor, to understand why some migraine sufferers associate some of their attacks with the inhalation of certain substances. These include tobacco smoke, paint, perfume, and house-dusts.

There are a number of types of hypersensitivity reaction, and one of these involves mast cell degranulation and the release of vasoactive amines. This release of vasoactive amines may provide the link between allergy and migraine, since the onset of a migraine attack is associated with an increase in vasoactive amine metabolism. Indeed, Grant (1979) considered that both immunological and non-immunological mechanisms may play a part in the pathogenesis of migraine caused by food intolerance. Although the immunological role may have been exaggerated in the past, there is little reason to dissent from this view.

An allergy can be defined as a hypersensitivity to a foreign body or antigen, which under suitable circumstances can stimulate a specific immune response with the production of antibodies. Immunoglobulin E (IgE) antibodies are specifically concerned in the immediate type of allergic reaction.

Using a radioallergosorbent test (RAST) for specific IgE antibody to foods, Monro *et al.* (1980) concluded that food allergy plays a part in migraine. Monro and colleagues investigated a number of foods including milk, cheese, egg, chocolate and wheat. However, the lack of information about controls and the caution with which the RAST should be interpreted makes it difficult to assess the results.

Other immunological abnormalities have also been looked for in migraine sufferers. The complement system comprises a system of serologically specific proteins present in fresh, normal serum, which are necessary for the death or lysis of cellular antigens in the present of antibody. In 1977 Lord *et al.* looked for evidence of complement activation related to migraine attacks and found significant reductions in C3 and C4 during headache periods. They considered that complement activation could explain many of the previously demonstrated phenomena occurring in migraine. Lord and Duckworth (1978) extended these studies using a C1q precipitation technique and found a significant correlation between the presence of immune complexes and the onset of headache in sera from migraine patients without prodromal symptoms.

In 1980, Sovak *et al.* reported on their investigations into C1 inhibitor levels in migraine subjects and controls. They found no significant differences and concluded that they had not identified an immunological defect in the pathophysiology of migraine. Similarly Moore *et al.* (1980) found no evidence of hypocomplementaemia, hypergammaglobulinaemia or evidence of increased levels of immune complexes in patients during the migraine episode as contrasted to the headache-free period.

Behan *et al.* (1980) studied 40 patients with migraine. They measured complement components C1q, C4, C3, C7, and Factor B, together with the conversion products of C3 and Factor B. CH_{50} units were also estimated and anticomplementary activity was assayed. No abnormalities were detected in any of the patients either in an attack or during a remission. Their results did not confirm that complement activation plays a role in migraine headache.

Since both immune factors and multifactorial inheritance have been proposed in migraine, O'Neill *et al.* (1979) have examined whether or not there is an association between HLA antigens of the major histocompatibility complex and migraine. They were unable to confirm this in their tests.

It would therefore seem that it is unusual for allergic reactions to trigger attacks of migraine or other types of headache, and migraine which owes its origin to allergy alone must be uncommon. Indeed, in the vast majority of cases, it is now clear that the induction of migraine by food has other explanations.

MECHANISM OF MIGRAINE

Why do certain articles of food precipitate migraine in some sufferers? We have to recognize that even in dietary migraine sufferers all of their attacks are unlikely to be the result of dietary factors alone. While there are some migraine sufferers who very often develop an attack after they have eaten a particular food, e.g. chocolate, in the majority of sufferers the precipitants of migraine are cumulative in effect.

The most common precipitant of migraine is stress. In this context the term stress includes such states as anger, excitement, fatigue, and exertion. Hormonal changes and hypoglycaemia can also act as precipitants. The common link between all these precipitants is that they result in changes in vasoactive amine metabolism. In 1961 Sicuteri *et al.* first reported an increase in the excretion of vanilmandelic acid (VMA) during migraine attacks. VMA excretion reflects, at least in part, catecholamine metabolism in the body. In 1961 Sicuteri reported an increase in the excretion of 5-hydroxyindoleacetic acid during migraine attacks. This reflects an increase in 5-hydroxytryptamine (5HT) metabolism in the body. Plasma 5HT levels rise at the onset of a migraine attack and fall during the attack (Curran *et al.*, 1965; Anthony *et al.*, 1967).

All the 5HT present in blood is contained in the platelets. Fozard (1981) has collated the results of nine studies and calculated that the mean fall of total platelet 5HT levels during an attack of migraine is 36 per cent.

Not only 5HT but all the vasoactive monoamines present in food such as tyramine and BPEA are broken down in the body by the enzyme MAO. A deficiency in platelet MAO during attacks has been reported (Sandler *et al.*, 1970; Glover *et al.*, 1977).

An increase in platelet aggregation in migraine sufferers was first reported by Hilton and Cumings in 1971. The fact that so many of the changes associated with migraine can be linked with changes in platelet behaviour led to the hypothesis that migraine is a blood disorder and due to a primary abnormality of platelet function (Hanington, 1978). Thus the development of a migraine attack can be illustrated diagrammatically as shown in Figure 2.

The symptoms occurring during the prodromal phase of classical migraine closely resemble the symptoms reported in transient ischaemic attacks. They could be due to cerebral ischaemia resulting from vasoconstriction with or

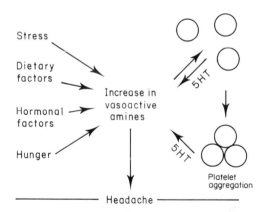

FIGURE 2   Vasoactive amines and migraine

without the temporary blockage of small vessels by platelet aggregates. Spontaneous aggregation and platelet adhesion are increased at all times in migraine sufferers (Deshmukh and Meyer, 1977; Hanington *et al.*, 1981).

During an attack of migraine changes occur in the size of cerebral blood vessels. The cerebral circulation is singularly sensitive to the effects of 5HT. It is of major importance that the platelets of migraine sufferers show significant changes in 5HT release and that these differences are closely related to the timing of a migraine attack (Hanington *et al.*, 1981).

Although there is a fall of approximately 36 per cent in total platelet 5HT concentration in migraine platelets during an attack, by the end of an attack the platelet 5HT levels have returned to normal and do not differ from those of control platelets. However, significant changes in the amounts of 5HT that are released from migraine platelets are detected in relation to the timing of an attack. Thus immediately after an attack and for at least 3 days after an attack, the 5HT released from migraine platelets is small. Then there is a slow, steady build-up of potential 5HT release and midway between two attacks a significant increase is detectable. At the onset of an attack there is a highly significant release of 5HT from the platelets. Then the whole cycle begins again as illustrated in Figure 3.

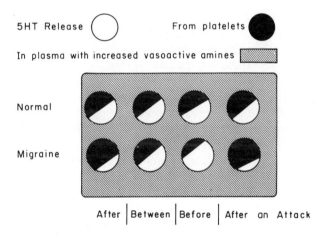

FIGURE 3   Platelet release of 5-hydroxytryptamine (5HT) in relationship to migraine attacks

Thus migraine attacks occur when two states coincide, namely a significant increase in plasma vasoactive amines and the ability of the migraine platelets to release highly significant amounts of 5HT.

While it is of major importance, 5HT is not the only substance released from platelets during a migraine attack. Other substances such as adenosine triphosphate, adenosine diphosphate, prostaglandins, and kinins are also involved. It is highly likely that these also take part in the complex vascular and biochemical changes occurring at the time of an attack.

Thus migraine appears to be due to a primary abnormality of platelet behaviour. This explains the frequently familial incidence of migraine, since platelet behaviour is genetically controlled. It also explains why the incidence of migraine is affected by the use of steroid hormones since these have a marked effect on platelet behaviour and in particular on 5HT receptors in platelets (Somerville, 1972; Peters *et al.*, 1979). Hanington *et al.* (1982) have found that the use of oral contraception can produce changes in platelet behaviours which are found in non-pill-taking migraine patients. It also explains why migraine has been reported as occurring for the first time in patients with platelet disorders, e.g. thrombocytopaenic purpura. In these patients attacks occurred when there was a sudden rapid fall in platelet count at a time when a sudden release of 5HT would have taken place (Damasio and Beck, 1978). In keeping with this, my colleague Dr John Amess and I have been looking after a migraine patient whose headaches greatly increased in frequency and severity as she developed an increasingly severe thrombocythaemia.

CONCLUSION

There is little doubt that certain foods can play a part in precipitating some attacks of migraine in some sufferers. When patients are questioned in a migraine clinic about possible precipitants of their attacks roughly one in three mention specific foods. However, claims that food factors play a major role in migraine (Dalton, 1975; Grant, 1979) need very careful interpretation. When dealing with individual patients it is important not to influence them into thinking that foods are concerned in precipitating their attacks. Since the tyramine studies were first reported in 1967 so much has been written about the possible relationship between substances like chocolate and migraine that it would no longer be easy to obtain an unbiased assessment of the position in Britain today. It is generally recognized that about 30 per cent of migraine sufferers respond, at least for a while, to placebo therapy. Stress is a major precipitant of migraine attacks and the knowledge that sympathy and interest are being shown will in itself be of help to most patients.

The cumulative effect of the various precipitants of migraine can be observed clinically. Thus a tired, anxious migraine sufferer who has missed a meal and eaten a bar of chocolate is then more likely to develop an attack than at a time when only one of these factors is operating. Even so, an attack of migraine may not be inevitable. When patients were tested with tyramine it soon became apparent that tyramine should not be given during the 3 days after an attack, as another attack was unlikely to occur. The reason for this refractory period has now been explained by the discovery of the recurring cycle of 5HT release that takes place in the migraine platelet (Hanington *et al.*, 1981).

The first essential in the treatment of migraine is that every sufferer should be considered and treated on an individual basis. There is no uniform therapy for this disorder. A careful assessment of the history and possible precipitants in the patient concerned must be followed by a careful clinical examination. Factors such as hypertension can contribute to the severity of attacks.

The patient should be given an explanation of why attacks of migraine occur, and adequate time for discussion is essential, particularly at the first consultation. All the common precipitants of migraine should be considered in turn. In this context such factors as the influence of oral contraception can be considered. Even in patients who recognize no dietary precipitants it is worth having an initial trial period of 6 weeks during which the sufferer excludes the common dietary precipitants such as cheese, chocolate, alcohol, and citrus fruits from the diet. The position can then be reassessed in the light of the results.

When patients appreciate the cumulative effect of the precipitants of migraine they are often able to do a great deal to help themselves. As far as diet is concerned it may prove necessary to exclude chocolate, cheese, and alcohol from the diet but more extreme measures are rarely needed. A woman who often has a migraine attack at the beginning of a menstrual period may benefit from avoiding chocolate, cheese, and alcohol only in the 5 days before her period is due.

In the initial stages of treatment it is helpful if the patient keeps a record of attacks, noting possible precipitants and any other relevant factors. A gradual picture will then emerge on which longer-term therapy can be based.

ACKNOWLEDGEMENTS

The author is grateful to the Wellcome Trustees for supporting her research.

REFERENCES

Anthony, M., and Lance, J. W. (1971). Histamine and serotonin in cluster headache. *Arch. Neurol.*, **25**, 225–31.

Anthony, M., Hinterberg, H., and Lance, J. W. (1967). Plasma serotonin in migraine and stress. *Arch. Neurol.*, **16**, 544–52.

Anthony, M., Lord, G. D. A., and Lance, J. W. (1978). Controlled trials of cimetidine in migraine and cluster headache. *Headache*, **18**, 261–4.

Balyeat, R. M., and Rinkel, H. J. (1931). Further studies in allergic migraine. *Ann. Int. Med.*, **5**, 713.

Behan, W. M. H., Behan, P. O., and Durward, W. F. (1980). Complement studies in migraine. *Headache*, **21**, 55–7.

Bethune, H. C., Burrell, R. H., and Culpan, R. H. (1963). Headache associated with monoamine oxidase inhibitors. *Lancet*, **2**, 1233.

Blackwell, B. (1963). Hypertensive crisis due to monoamine oxidase inhibitors, *Lancet*, **2**, 849–51.

Blackwell, B., and Mabbitt, L. A. (1965). The tyramine content of cheese and its relationship to the hypertensive crisis after monoamine oxidase inhibition, *Lancet*, **1**, 938-40.

Blackwell, B., and Marley, E. (1964). Interactions between cheese and monoamine oxidase inhibitors in rats and cats. *Lancet*, **1**, 530-1.

Blackwell, B., and Marley, E. (1966). Interactions of cheese and of its constituents with monoamine oxidase inhibitors. *Br. J. Pharmacol.*, **26**, 120-41.

Blackwell, B., Marley, E., Price, J., and Taylor, D. (1967). Hypertensive interactions between monoamine oxidase inhibitors and foodstuffs. *Br. J. Psychiatry*, **113**, 349-65.

Blackwell, B., Mabbitt, L. A., and Marley, E. (1969). Histamine and tyramine content of yeast products. *J. Food. Sci.*, **34**, 47-51.

Bonnett, G. F., and Nepveux, P. (1971). Les migraines tyraminiques, *Sem. Hôp. Paris*, **47**, 2441-5.

Colldahl, H. (1965). Allergy and certain diseases in relation to the digestive tract. *Acta Allergol. (Kbh)*, **20**, 84.

Curran, D. A., Hinterberger, H., and Lance, J. W. (1965). Total plasma serotonin, 5-hydroxyindole acetic acid and *p*-hydroxy-*m*-methoxymandelic acid excretion in normal and migranous subjects. *Brain*, **88**, 997-1010.

Dalton, Katharina (1975). Food intake prior to a migraine attack—study of 2213 spontaneous attacks. *Headache*, **15** (3), 188-93.

Damasio, H., and Beck, D. (1978). Migraine, thrombocytopenia and serotonin metabolism. *Lancet*, **1**, 240-2.

Deshmukh, S. B., and Meyer, J. S. (1977). Cyclic changes in platelet dynamics and the pathogenesis and prophylaxis of migraine. *Headache*, **17**, 101-8.

Evans, C. S., Bell, E. A., and Stewart Johnson, E. (1979). *N*-Methyltyramine. A biologically active amine in acacia seeds. *Phytochemistry*, **18**, 2022-3.

Fothergill, John (1784). *Medical Observations and Enquiries*, **6**, 103-37.

Fozard, J. R. (1981). Serotonin, migraine, and platelets. *Progress in Pharmacology*, Vol. 4. *Drugs and Platelets* (eds P. A. Van Zweiten and E. Schönbaum). Gustav Fischer, Verlag, Stuttgart.

Froeberg, J., Carlson, L. A., Karlsson, C. G., Levi, L., and Seeman, K. (1969). Effects of coffee on catecholamine excretion and plasma lipids. In: *Coffein und andere Methylxanthine* (eds F. Heim and H. P. Ammon). Schattauerverlag, Stuttgart New York, pp.65-73.

Ghose, K., Coppen, A., and Carroll, D. (1977). Intravenous tyramine response in migraine before and during treatment with indoramin. *Br. Med. J.*, **1**, 1191-3.

Glover, V., Sandler, M., Grant, E., Rose, F. C., Orton, D., Wilkinson, M., and Stevens, D. (1977). Transitory decrease in platelet monoamine oxidase activity during migraine attacks. *Lancet*, **1**, 391-3.

Granerus, G. (1968). Effects of oral histamine, histidine and diet on urinary excretion of histamine, methylhistamine and 1-methyl-4-imidazole acetic acid in man. *Scand. J. Clin. Lab. Invest.*, **22** (suppl. 104), 49-58.

Grant, E. C. G. (1979). Food allergies and migraine. *Lancet*, **1**, 966-8.

Hanington, Edda (1967). Preliminary report on tyramine headache. *Br. Med. J.*, **2**, 550-1.

Hanington, Edda (1970). Migraine. *Trans. Med. Soc. London*, **87**, 32-9.

Hanington, Edda (1978). Migraine: a blood disorder? *Lancet*, **2**, 501-3.

Hanington, Edda, and Harper, A. M. (1968). The role of tyramine in the aetiology of migraine and related studies of the cerebral and extracanial circulations. *Headache*, **8**, 84-97.

Hanington, E., Horn, M., and Wilkinson, M. (1970). Further observations on the effects of tyramine. In: *Background to Migraine*, 3rd Migraine Symposium (ed. A. L. Cochrane). Heinemann Medical, London, pp.113–19.

Hanington, Edda, Jones, R. J., Amess, J. A. L., and Wachowicz, B. (1981). Migraine —a platelet disorder. *Lancet*, 2, 721–3.

Hanington, E., Jones, R. J., and Amess, J. A. L. (1982). Platelet aggregation in response to SHT in migraine patients taking oral contraceptives. *Lancet*, 1, 967–8.

Henderson, W. R., and Raskin, N. H. (1972). 'Hot dog' headache: individual susceptibility to nitrite. *Lancet*, 2, 1162–3.

Hilton, B. P., and Cumings, J. N. (1971). An assessment of platelet aggregation induced by 5-hydroxytryptamine. *J. Clin. Pathol.*, 24, 250–8.

Horton, B. T., McClean, A. R., and Craig, W. M. A. (1939). A new syndrome of vascular headache, results of treatment with histamine: preliminary report. *Mayo Clin. Proc.*, 14, 257–60.

Howitz, D., Lovenberg, W., Engelmann, K., and Sjoerdsma, A. (1964). Monoamine oxidase inhibitors, tyramine and cheese. *J. Am. Med. Assoc.*, 188, 1108.

Kallos, P., and Kallos-Deffner, L. (1955). Allergy and migraine. *Int. Arch. Allergy*, 7, 367.

Kudrow, Lee (1980). *Cluster Headache: mechanisms and management*. Oxford University Press, Oxford, p.37.

Littlewood, J., Glover, V., and Sandler, M. (1982). Platelet phenolsulphotransferase deficiency in dietary migraine. *Lancet*, 1, 983–6.

Liveing, Edward (1873). *On Megrim, Sick-Headache and some Allied Disorders.* J. & A. Churchill, London.

Lord, G. D. A., and Duckworth, J. W. (1978). Complement and immune complex studies in migraine. *Headache*, 18, 255–60.

Lord, G. D. A., Duckworth, J. W., and Charlesworth, J. A. (1977). Complement activation in migraine. *Lancet*, 1, 781–2.

Maxwell, H. (1965). Migraine and allergy. *Practitioner*, 195, 803–8.

Mayer, K., and Pause, G. (1973). Nicht fluechtige biogene. Amine in Wein. *Travaux de Chimie Alimentaire et d'Hygiene*, 64, 171–9.

Mayer, K., Pause, G., and Vetsch, U. (1971). Histaminbildung während der Weinbereitung. *Travaux de Chimie alimentaire et d'Hygiene*, 62 (4), 397–406.

Monro, J., Carini, C., Brostoff, J., and Zilkha, K. (1980). Food allergy in migraine. *Lancet*, 2, 1–4.

Moore, T. L., Ryan, R. E., Pohl, D. A., Roodman, S. T., and Ryan, R. E., Jr. (1980). Immunoglobulin, complement and immune complex levels during a migraine attack. *Headache*, 20, 9–12.

O'Neill, B. P., Kapur, J. J., and Good, A. E. (1979). H.L.A. antigens in migraine. *Headache*, 19, 71–3.

Paul, A. A., and Southgate, D. A. T. (1978). *McCance and Widdowson's—The Composition of Foods*. HMSO, London; Elsevier/North Holland Biomedical Press, Amsterdam.

Peters, J. R., Martin, E. J., and Grahame-Smith, D. G. (1979). Effect of oral contraceptives on platelet noradrenaline and 5-hydroxytryptamine receptors and aggregation. *Lancet*, 2, 933–6.

Raskin, N. H., and Knittle, S. C. (1976). Ice cream headache and orthostatic symptoms in patients with migraine. *Headache*, 16, 222–5.

Ryan, R. E. (1974). A clinical study of tyramine as an etiological factor in migraine. *Headache*, 14, 43–8.

Sandler, M., Youdim, M. B. H., Southgate, J., and Hanington, E. (1970). The role of tyramine in migraine: some possible biochemical mechanisms. In: *Background to Migraine*—3rd Migraine Symposium (ed. A. L. Cochrane). Heinemann Medical, London, pp.103–12.

Sandler, M., Youdin, M. B. H., and Hanington, E. (1974). A phenylethylamine oxidising defect in migraine. *Nature*, **250**, 335–7.

Schaumberg, H. H., Byck, R., Gerstl, R., and Mashman, J. H. (1969). Monosodium L-glutamate: its pharmacology and role in the Chinese restaurant syndrome. *Science*, **163**, 826–8.

Schwartz, M. (1952). Is migraine an allergic disease? *J. Allergy*, **23**, 426.

Schweitzer, J. W., Friedhoff, A. J., and Schwartz, R. (1975). Chocolate, betaphenylethylamine and migraine re-examined. *Nature*, **257**, 256–7.

Selbach, H. (1973). Coffein, Kaffee, Kopfschmerz und Migraene. *Med. Klin.*, **68**, 642–8.

Sen, N. P. (1969). Analyses and significance of tyramine in foods. *J. Food Sci.*, **34**, 22.

Sever, P. S. (1979). False transmitters and migraine. *Lancet*, **1**, 333.

Sicuteri, F., Testi, A., and Anselmi, B. (1961). Biochemical investigations in headache: increase in the hydroxyindole acid excretion during migraine attacks. *Int. Arch. Allergy Appl. Immunol.*, **19**, 55–8.

Sjaastad, O., and Sjaastad, O. V. (1977). Urinary histamine excretion in migraine and cluster headache. *J. Neurol.*, **216**, 91–104.

Smith, I., Kellow, A. K., and Hanington, E. (1970). A clinical and biochemical correlation between tyramine and migraine headache. *Headache*, **10**, 43–52.

Somerville, B. W. (1972). The influence of progesterone and oestradiol upon migraine. *Headache*, **12**, 93–102.

Southgate, J., Grant, E. C. G., Pollard, W., Pryse Davies, J., and Sandler, M. (1968). Cyclical variations in endometrial monoamine oxidase. Correlation of histochemical and quantitative biochemical assays. *Biochem. Pharmacol.*, **17**, 721.

Sovak, M., Kunzel, M., Dalessio, D. J., and Lang, J. H. (1980). C-1 Inhibitor levels in migraineurs and normals. *Headache*, **20**, 132–3.

Thompson, R. H. S., and Tickner, A. (1949). Observations on the monoamine oxidase activity of placenta and uterus. *Biochem. J.*, **45**, 125.

Thompson, R. H. S., and Tickner, A. (1951). The occurrence and distribution of monoamine oxidase in blood vessels. *J. Physiol.*, **115**, 34.

Udenfried, S., Lovenberg, W., and Sjoerdsma, A. (1959). Physiologically active amines in common fruits and vegetables. *Arch. Biochem.*, **85**, 487.

Unger, A. H., and Unger, L. (1952). Migraine is an allergic disease. *J. Allergy*, **23**, 429.

Walker, Vera B. (1963). Allergy in migraine. *J. Coll. Gen. Pract.*, **6** (suppl. No. 4), 21.

Clinical Reactions to Food
Edited by M. H. Lessof
© 1983 John Wiley & Sons Ltd.

Coeliac Disease, Inflammatory Bowel Disease, and Food Intolerance

W. T. Cooke

*Honorary Consultant Physician and Gastroenterologist,
The General Hospital, Birmingham*

and

G. K. T. Holmes

*Consultant Physician and Gastroenterologist,
The Derbyshire Royal Infirmary, Derby;
Clinical Tutor, the University of Nottingham, Nottingham*

The fact has been established that wheat protein — a component of a common foodstuff, bread — can be responsible for the ill-health of a group of patients (Dicke, 1950) and can produce histological changes in the intestinal tract. This finding initiated a fresh approach to many medical problems and was a powerful stimulus for research into intestinal and nutritional disorders. The concept is now applicable much more widely than only to the role of gluten in coeliac disease.

COELIAC DISEASE

Historical perspective

Samuel Gee's classical description of the coeliac affection pointed out that 'the allowance of farinaceous food must be small: highly starched food, rice, sago, corn-flour are unfit', and concluded with that much quoted comment, 'if the patient can be cured at all, it must be by means of diet' (Gee, 1888). In 1914,

Poynton and his colleagues noted that bread and butter could not be added to the diet of one of their coeliac children without causing a relapse in the symptoms. In 1918, Still, in his Lumleian lectures stated that 'one form of starch which seems particularly liable to aggravate symptoms is bread'. Howland (1921) in America wrote that 'of all the elements of the food, carbohydrate is the one which must be excluded rigorously', and concluded, 'bread, cereals and potato are the last articles that can be allowed'. Parsons (1932) recognized that coeliac disease did not occur in infants still being breast-fed. In 1947, Andersen suggested that both cereals and starch were responsible for the harmful effect upon fat absorption, and Sheldon in 1949 noted that steatorrhoea was reduced when foods containing flour were excluded. As Dicke (1950) pointed out, the solution was very close. In Holland during World War II, contrary to expectation, coeliac children had done much better when flour had been scarce. Dicke demonstrated that the removal of wheat and rye flours from the diet caused the symptoms and signs of coeliac disease to disappear. Subsequently, in a classic series of experiments, Van de Kamer *et al.* (1953) demonstrated that gluten and in particular one of its components, gliadin, was the toxic factor in wheat. They recommended the exclusion of wheat, barley, oats, and rye from the diet.

Research over the past 30 years has aimed at isolating the specific component of wheat which is toxic to coeliac patients. The gluten factor, obtained by various methods of digestion, is a mixture of amino acids, glycopeptides, acidic peptides, dialysable and non-dialysable peptides, and enzymes with differing properties according to their basic protein chains and the attacked side-chains of non-protein conjugates, all differing in their chemical and physiochemical properties. It is perhaps not surprising that identification still eludes us. Nevertheless, a vast amount of information on the clinical manifestations, the immunological responses of the patient, and the constitutional background of the disorder has been amassed but has raised more questions than answers.

Definition

Definition of a disease is necessary for analysis and evaluation of clinical data and research, and requires revision periodically as new knowledge becomes available. Definitions of coeliac disease, or gluten enteropathy, revolve around the changes in the jejunal mucosa following gluten challenge or withdrawal and the associated clinical reactions. From a practical point of view, diagnosis in the majority of patients is relatively simple and made on the presence of a characteristic flat jejunal biopsy and a satisfactory clinical response to gluten withdrawal. However, there remain a number of patients in whom the diagnosis is not easy and with increasing knowledge of disorders of the small intestine definition has, if anything, become more difficult. Most workers require a flat jejunal biopsy, but others only an abnormal mucosa. It would appear logical to assume that if gluten withdrawal can lead to reversion of the mucosa to normal, then all stages from apparent normality to a flat biopsy should be found in patients with coeliac disease on a normal diet. There is evidence to suggest that this is indeed the case. Patients with dermatitis herpetiformis and apparently normal jejunal mucosa can be made to produce a flat biopsy on loading with gluten (Weinstein, 1974). Children taking a gluten-containing diet and with morphologically normal small bowel mucosa have subsequently developed a flat biopsy (Egan-Mitchell et al., 1981). In addition, relatives of coeliac probands show an increased incidence of mild abnormalities of their mucosa, an excess of HLA B8 antigens (Stokes et al., 1976) and IgA antireticulin antibodies (Mallas et al., 1977); they too may produce an abnormal mucosa on increasing their gluten intake (Doherty and Barry, 1981). There are difficulties in the interpretation of gluten challenge. Good clinical response may take place without morphological improvement of the mucosa, and little or no clinical response in the presence of excellent morphological recovery (Cooke and Holmes, 1977). The morphological response may take months or even years to develop (McNicholl et al., 1979), though the majority show change within a few weeks. Undoubtedly, the age, immunological status, endocrinological maturity, and genetic make-up of patients influence their response to gluten. A positive gluten challenge can only demonstrate that a patient has coeliac disease whilst a negative result cannot exclude it. In summary, nearly all patients will have a flat biopsy and most will show clear-cut improvement on a gluten-free diet. Exceptions to these generalizations will continue to surface and provoke argument regarding their relationship to coeliac disease. For the moment then, an all-enveloping definition is not possible.

Sex and age incidence

This disorder is usually considered to be more common in women than men. Consideration of 18 reported series, covering 2600 patients, showed that the ratio of women to men was 1.26 to 1. The age of onset of symptoms bears little upon the age of presentation or of diagnosis. Our oldest patient presented at the age of 84 years, though with symptoms for more than 20 years. Now at the age of 90 she is an expert cook of gluten-free diets. There are certain times of life when the disorder is more likely to appear. One about which there is little doubt is the period following the introduction of gluten to the diet so that most child coeliacs are diagnosed before the age of 2 years (McNeish and Anderson, 1974). It is also claimed that there is a peak incidence in women in the fourth decade and in the sixth and seventh decades for men (Swinson and Levi, 1980). The increased incidence of coeliac disease during the 1950s and 1960s has been attributed to the practice of introducing cereals at an increasingly early age, often at the age of only 4–6 weeks, whilst the apparent decrease since 1974 has been ascribed to the reversal of this practice to introduction at not less than 6 months.

Racial and geographical incidence

In many respects, coeliac disease can be regarded as a disorder of western Europe and related to the cereal-consuming habits of these countries. The incidence is probably greater than the reported figures at present suggest. Thus, in England and Scotland, the incidence has been calculated to lie between 1 in 1100 and 1 in 4000 (Carter et al., 1959; Davidson and Fountain, 1950). In Ireland it may be as high as 1 in 303 (Mylotte et al., 1973). The incidence in Sweden, Switzerland, Norway, and France is somewhat similar to that in the United Kingdom, with Austria having an incidence similar to Ireland. Coeliac disease is known to occur in Brazil, Argentina, South Africa, and Australasia, though probably only in those of European stock. However, it has been diagnosed in Indians, Cubans, Mexicans, Arabs, and in Arab-Negro stock. A clue may lie in the observation that in India, coeliac disease is found in the wheat-eating areas of Bengal and the Punjab and not in the rice-eating areas of southern India (Misra et al., 1966; Walia et al., 1966). There are difficulties in ascribing the incidence to dietary habits only, for the frequency of clinical recognition of coeliac disease in the United States appears to be considerably less than that in Western Europe. This is in spite of having a large ethnic population derived from Europe, being the largest cereal producer in the world and with a similar incidence of coeliac disease amongst first-degree relatives to that found in Europe (MacDonald et al., 1965). There are, however, no adequate figures of the incidence in America on which to base valid comment. It has been suggested that this apparent anomaly may be due to the type of wheat grown, which might lack the toxic component (Ciclitira et al., 1980; Kasarda et al., 1976). Improved diagnostic methods and follow-up of patients in the future may provide an explanation.

The nature of the toxic factor

Wheat flour is made up of starch (70–75 per cent), proteins (7–15 per cent), lipids (1–2 per cent), water (14 per cent), and small amounts of other substances such as salts and nucleic acids (Ewart, 1970). Approximately 90 per cent of wheat protein is gluten, which itself is a heterogeneous group of proteins which have not yet been completely characterized. When treated with 70 per cent alcohol, the soluble fraction, gliadin, is removed, leaving behind the insoluble fraction glutenin, the component responsible for the viscoelastic properties characteristic of dough. The gliadin fraction with a high content of glutamine and proline is also complex. When only a single wheat variety is used as a source, there are more than 40 different components, artificially divided into four groups α, β, γ and ω gliadins on the basis of their electrophoretic mobilities. The molecular weights may lie between 30,000 and 50,000, but there are considerable difficulties in isolating pure components for assessment. The concept has developed that a carbohydrate side-chain may be responsible for toxicity (Phelan *et al.*, 1977). An exceptionally proline-rich protein, moderately rich in glutamine and glutamic acid, has been extracted from the acid alcohol-soluble fraction of gluten. It is claimed to act as a lectin by reacting with genetically incomplete glycosyl chains on the proteins of the intestinal mucosa (Douglas, 1976; Weiser and Douglas, 1976). Peptides derived from gluten have also been isolated in brain tissue, which may have some relevance to the mood and mental changes encountered in coeliac disease (Zioudrou *et al.*, 1979). Flour derived from cereals other than wheat is also toxic. That from rye is of similar toxicity to wheat flour, but that from barley and oats is less so. The amount of gliadin derived from oats is only a sixth of that from wheat. Maize and rice do not appear to be damaging. The average daily intake of gluten for the British adult has been estimated at 7 g. According to the Food Advisory Bureau, one thick slice of either white or wholemeal bread contains approximately 1 g of gluten. There is, however, considerable divergence of opinion as to the amounts of gluten found in foods and the daily diet. Gluten-free flour has for its basis wheat starch which is obtained by removing gluten from wheat flour in a washing process. This wheat starch should contain less than 0.5 per cent protein if it is to be considered non-toxic to coeliacs. Unfortunately, in commercial practice, it may contain greater amounts of protein and still be labelled starch; and though designated gluten-free, it may be toxic. Other sources of hidden gluten are textured vegetable protein, vegetable protein, and cereal binders, which may or may not be gluten-free.

The clinical presentation

Since the classic description by Gee (1888), the many reports of the clinical aspects of coeliac disease have tended to concentrate on the grosser manifestations of the disorder. Patients may still present with severe illness, but it is evident that many have virtually no symptoms or at the most, completely non-specific complaints. Such patients will only be diagnosed as a result of greater awareness of the significance of minor abnormalities encountered in the haematological and biochemical profiles. These relatively asymptomatic patients are still at risk of developing the serious complications of coeliac disease.

Symptoms can tentatively be divided into those which are directly due to the effects of gluten and those which result from the damage to the small intestinal mucosa caused by gluten. Obviously, some could result for either reason.

Symptoms probably due to the direct effect of gluten

The symptoms directly due to gluten will readily be recognized in infants, for example on weaning with cereals, or in older subjects treated by a gluten-free diet who are challenged with gluten. Thus, in infancy, anorexia, failure to thrive, profuse vomiting without effort, abdominal pain severe enough to mimic intestinal obstruction, abdominal distension, and diarrhoea all occur. Some adults will react merely by feeling unwell for a few hours or even a few weeks. In the majority, the common symptoms are malaise, nausea, anorexia, abdominal distension, and some looseness of stool. A few will have no clinical symptoms at all despite the fact that they will produce definite histological change in their jejunal mucosa in the weeks or months following the reintroduction of gluten to the diet. Rarely, the response to gluten can be violent. 'Gluten shock' was described by Van de Kamer *et al.* (1953):

> One of the patients with coeliac disease happened to show an abnormally violent reaction to the administration of any form of wheat—three to six hours after administration, severe abdominal pain, vomiting, pallor and sometimes even slight shock—even a small piece of rusk or biscuit caused vomiting, abdominal pain etc. within a few hours.

Menstruation and fertility

Disturbances in menstruation and fertility are a common cause for complaint and are largely relieved by exclusion of gluten from the diet. Thus, in untreated coeliac disease, the menarche is significantly delayed and the menopause significantly earlier than in treated coeliacs or the normal population (Ferguson *et al.*, 1982). Episodes of amenorrhoea or oligomenorrhoea are frequent. Though many coeliac patients have children, as a group they are relatively infertile and a gluten-free diet may result in conception relatively rapidly. The mechanism by which gluten exerts these effects is unknown.

Growth

Short stature is another cause for complaint (Groll *et al.*, 1980) which appears to be related to a direct effect of gluten, and a return to normal growth rate is one criterion by which the efficacy of treatment can be judged. Tall patients, however, do occur. Three of our male coeliac patients were more than 6 feet tall (183 cm) and two of the women more than 5 feet 10 inches (178 cm).

Mental change

The mood and mental changes that follow the exclusion of gluten from the diet of an untreated coeliac patient are well known and form a characteristic symptomatology (Paulley, 1959). Depression, in particular, has been commented upon and has been considered a prominent feature of childhood coeliac disease (Sheldon, 1959). We encountered 25 women and 6 men amongst 314 biopsy-proven coeliacs who needed treatment for depression. Three made suicidal attempts, one of which was successful. Of interest are the terms that have been applied to these mental disturbances in the untreated patient—schizoid, depressive, querulous, irritable, obsessional, neurotic, paranoid, and delusional (Paulley, 1959; Kazer, 1961; Townley and Anderson, 1967).

Dementia and schizophrenia

Actual organic dementia is a significant feature of some patients. Degenerative changes are readily demonstrable in the cerebrum and other areas of the brain (Cooke and Smith, 1966). The mental changes appear to be arrested on withdrawal of gluten from the diet (Cooke, 1976). Schizophrenia in our series of over 400 coeliacs had an incidence of at least 10 per 1000: an incidence as high at 37 per 1000 has been quoted, compared with an incidence of 2.3–4.7 per 1000 in the general population. A relationship between schizophrenia and coeliac disease has been suggested (Dohan, 1966) though an Irish study could not confirm this (Stevens et al., 1977). However, the response of lymphocytes from a group of schizophrenics, to stimulation with subfractions of gluten was comparable to that found in untreated coeliac disease (Ashkenazi et al., 1979). It is probable that exclusion of gluten from the diet of schizophrenics is beneficial (Dohan and Glasberger, 1973) and in practice it can greatly improve the mental state of coeliac patients who are also schizophrenic.

The incidence of schizophrenia in the population has been correlated with the geographical incidence of cereal consumption, the greatest incidence being in those areas of predominant wheat and rye consumption, and the lowest in the areas of sorghan and maize (Dohan, 1966). Disturbances in biopterin metabolism may be relevant in the aetiology of these mental disturbances. Crithidia factor, a co-factor in neural tissues for the hydroxylation of tyrosine to dihydrophenylanine in the synthesis of amine transmitters—dopamine, noradrenaline and adrenaline—(Smith et al., 1975; Leeming et al., 1976) is present in significantly low levels in patients with senile dementia, schizophrenia, and untreated coeliac disease (Leeming and Blair, 1980). Peptides derived from gluten, and resistant to trypsin and chymotrypsin, can be detected in brain tissue and may be particularly relevant in this respect (Zioudrou et al., 1979).

Aphthous ulceration

Aphthous stomatitis is relatively common in coeliac disease as it is in the general population. It may precede the more obvious manifestations of coeliac disease by many years (Ferguson *et al.*, 1976). It appears to be related to gluten ingestion since a gluten-free diet results in the disappearance of the ulcers. Though there may be many factors and possibly other foodstuffs, the ability of gluten to produce these lesions in some non-coeliac patients has been clearly demonstrated (Wray, 1981), though the mechanism is by no means clear.

Symptoms probably due to the gluten-damaged mucosa

Other common symptoms may be due to the direct effect of gluten on the relevant tissue but in our opinion are more likely to be due mainly to the damage caused to the small intestine by gluten, i.e. largely a secondary effect. Such damage affects the upper small intestine principally. Only rarely, in our experience of more than 40 post mortems, has the whole of the small intestine been affected. During life there is a depression of the mucosal enzymes such as the disaccharidases and peptidases of the upper intestinal tract and also changes in the gut hormones. Furthermore, the mucosal damage is associated with alteration in the intraluminal pH (Benn and Cooke, 1971) and that of the glycocalyx towards alkalinity (Lucas *et al.*, 1978), with the consequence that absorption of drugs and nutrients is considerably disrupted and, in the long term, making the development of deficiency states likely.

Bowel upset

Loose stools or diarrhoea are classical symptoms, though they may be absent in an appreciable number of patients. Clearly they may result from a direct reaction to gluten but in many patients other factors require consideration. One is the considerable reduction in absorptive surface that follows damage to the intestinal mucosa. Mere reduction in the length of the small intestine of a normal subject, to as little as 5 feet (150 cm), does not necessarily result in diarrhoea, as in one of our non-coeliac patients (Shenoi *et al.*, 1966). There is also an active secretion of sodium in the upper jejunum of coeliac patients (Fordtran *et al.*, 1967) for which compensation is made, in varying degrees, by increased absorption of water and electrolytes in the distal ileum (Schedl and Clifton, 1963). Presumably such a mechanism will play some part in the absence or otherwise of loose stools or diarrhoea. A further factor which is liable to cause diarrhoea is the loss of the mucosal enzymes resulting in lactose intolerance.

Electrolyte disturbance

As a result of diarrhoea, and even in coeliac patient with formed stools, there is an increased faecal loss of potassium (Cooke et al., 1953), the total body content of potassium is diminished (Blainey et al., 1954), and the consequences of electrolyte depletion, and zinc and magnesium loss, rapidly appear. Symptoms associated with these changes are lassitude, irritability, confusion, forgetfulness, ataxia, muscle weakness, muscle spasms, fits, loss of taste, and infertility.

Nocturnal diuresis

Nocturnal diuresis, a feature overlooked in the recent literature, may be sufficiently troublesome as to be the presenting symptom of coeliac disease. It is probably a reflection of electrolyte disturbance and depletion which may lead to the development of vacuolar tubular nephropathy and a complete reversal of the normal ratio of urinary excretion by day and night (Cooke, 1957). The disappearance of this symptom is a measure of the efficacy of treatment.

Three important complications—neuropathy, malignant disease, and disorders of bone metabolism—and one association/complication—dermatitis herpetiformis—are encountered which are partly due to the direct effect of gluten and partly result from the damaged small intestinal mucosa.

Neuropathy

Neuropathy tends to arise in patients of good general condition. Numbness, tingling, pain, weakness, and unsteady gait are some of the main symptoms that cause the patient to seek advice. Sensory ataxia rapidly becomes the most prominent symptom in nearly all patients. The legs are more affected than the arms, and attacks of unconsciousness are not uncommon (Cooke and Smith, 1966). It has been called 'progressive myeloradiculoneuropathy' and considered to be refractory to all medication (Sencer, 1957). In our experience, its incidence lies between 5 and 8 per cent of all cases followed for more than 10 years. It is not helped by a gluten-free diet or related to either folic acid or vitamin B_{12} deficiency. Pathologically, there are gross changes in the cerebrum, with atrophy and focal loss of neurons, with cortical or cerebellar atrophy in some patients, sufficiently marked to be recognized macroscopically. In the spinal cord, the lesions tend to be patchy and non-systematized and not those characteristically associated wtih subacute combined degeneration of the cord. In the peripheral nerves there is collateral branching and re-innervation together with diffuse swelling of the terminal axons which is most marked distally (Cooke et al., 1966). The cause of this neuropathy is not known. It may be due to a direct effect of gluten, but there is no improvement with exclusion of gluten from the diet. It might be secondary to changes in the neurotransmitters, or disturbance in tyrosine and pyridoxine metabolism already alluded to as one of the common metabolic defects in coeliac disease.

Malignancy

It is now well accepted that there is an increased incidence of malignancy in coeliac disease, both of carcinoma, particularly of the intestinal tract, and of reticulum cell sarcoma or malignant histiocytosis (Harris et al., 1967; Holmes et al., 1976; Isaacson and Wright, 1978). The increased incidence of carcinoma of the intestinal tract is not related to such factors as chronic iron deficiency or smoking. It could be related to the reduction of detoxicating enzymes in the mucosa which allows access of dietary carcinogens to the system (Wattenberg, 1966). The symptoms of carcinoma and the response to treatment are similar to those encountered in non-coeliac patients. Malignant lymphoma is characterized by ill-health, weight loss, abdominal pain, and diarrhoea. The diagnosis should be suspected in newly diagnosed coeliac patients who fail to respond to gluten withdrawal and also in those who deteriorate unaccountably after a period of excellent health on a gluten-free diet. Even when the diagnosis is suspected, it is difficult to confirm during life (Cooper et al., 1980a). There is at present no evidence that a gluten-free diet will prevent malignant complications. It may be that if a gluten-free diet does offer any protection against malignancy it will become apparent only in an analysis of a group of patients who have been on diet since childhood.

Bone disorder

Osteoporosis and osteomalacia have long been recognized as occurring commonly in coeliac disease. Amongst 118 coeliac patients investigated by bone biopsy, radiology, and biochemistry, 57 per cent had osteomalacia, two-thirds of whom had osteoporosis in addition, while seven had osteoporosis only. Symptoms tend to be insidious and include lassitude, bone pains, and 'joint' swellings in the rickets of childhood, and 'rheumatic pains' and altered gait in the adult. The altered gait is associated both with myopathy and with pseudofractures of the femoral neck or ramus pubis, and it is quite characteristic of osteomalacia. The proximal myopathy of vitamin D deficiency may occasionally be the first symptom leading to the diagnosis of coeliac disease (Cooke, 1976). At one time, cure was not considered possible unless gluten was removed from the diet, in the belief that gluten blocked the effect of vitamin D (Nassim et al., 1958; Moss et al., 1965). The principal reason, however, is the depressed absorption of vitamin D_3 (Melvin et al., 1970) brought about by alterations in pH of the microclimate of the small intestinal epithelium

(Hollander *et al.*, 1979). These abnormalities are reversed by withdrawal of gluten. Nevertheless, with or without gluten withdrawal, the administration of oral calciferol rarely rails to cure the osteomalacia even in the most severe cases. It must also be recognized that, occasionally, osteomalacia will make its appearance while patients are receiving a gluten-free diet, and also that this condition may sometimes resist therapy with calciferol and only respond to vitamin D_3 (Hepner *et al.*, 1978).

Dermatitis herpetiformis

Dermatitis herpetiformis is a papulovesicular rash which is usually located symmetrically on the knees, elbows, buttocks, face, trunk and sometimes within the mouth. The average case is relatively mild and in coeliac disease the lesions tend to be so few that their symmetrical distribution is difficult to appreciate. Abnormalities in the jejunal mucosa are found in 75 per cent of patients, with approximately equal proportions having a flat biopsy identical to that found in untreated coeliac disease, less severe defects, and only mild changes respectively. The remaining 25 per cent have apparently normal biopsies though there are increased lymphocyte numbers in the epithelium in some, which return to normal following gluten withdrawal (Fry *et al.*, 1972). A flat biopsy may result from gluten loading (Weinstein, 1974). Symptoms commonly encountered in patients with coeliac disease such as lassitude, diarrhoea, and abdominal distension are unusual in dermatitis herpetiformis, and symptomatic malabsorption is rarely encountered (Katz and Strober, 1978). Both conditions, however, have an increased incidence of HLA B8 but the diagnostic IgA deposits in the tips of the dermal papillae in dermatitis herpetiformis are not found in coeliac disease. The skin rash is benefited in over 90 per cent of patients by a gluten-free diet, irrespective of the state of the jejunal mucosa (Reunala *et al.*, 1977). The cause for the association between dermatitis herpetiformis, coeliac disease, and gluten is not known. The interesting patients, however, are those who fulfil the criteria for diagnosis, with IgA deposits in the skin, but who have completely normal jejunal biopsies and do not respond to a gluten-free diet. One can only speculate that some other toxic substance or food allergen may be involved. Sodium cromoglycate has no significant effect upon the lesions (Fry *et al.*, 1981).

Objective features

There is no one finding that is specific for the diagnosis of coeliac disease, either on physical examination or in the laboratory tests. However, the flat jejunal biopsy, with its mosaic pattern, absent villi, and cuboidal epithelium, is characteristic of the condition (Padykula *et al.*, 1961). The increased lymphocytic infiltration of the epithelium, and the increased plasma cell numbers in the lamina propria, appear to reflect an immunological response to antigens in the intestinal lumen.

A hypochromic, macrocytic anaemia of mild degree is a common finding in coeliac disease with at least half the patient having a haemoglobin greater than 12 g per cent when first seen. The principal cause is folate and iron deficiency. The serum levels of 5-methyltetrahydrofolic acid are usually reduced (Hoffbrand, 1974) because of poor absorption (Weir *et al.*, 1973), which appears largely due to the increased alkalinity of the surface microclimate. This increases the ionization of weak acids, which are thus unable to cross the negatively charged lipoid barrier of the glycocalyx (Blair and Matty, 1974; Kesavan and Noronha, 1978). Whether an active process of absorption plays any part is not yet proved. Iron deficiency is due to impaired absorption through the damaged mucosa and also to increased excretion of iron into the gut (Kosnai *et al.*, 1979). Thus, both deficiencies are essentially secondary to the damaged intestinal mucosa and are corrected by withdrawal of gluten from the diet. It must also be remembered that folic acid deficiency is responsible for some abnormalities in the mucosa such as villous shortening, increased crypt length, and megaloblastic change in the nuclei of the enterocytes and enteroblasts (Davidson and Townley, 1977). Deficiency of vitamin B_{12} is relatively uncommon, reflecting that the site of absorption, the distal ileum, is not usually affected in coeliac disease.

Hyposplenism with differing degrees of splenic atrophy is an important feature. Its presence can be suspected from the presence of Howell-Jolly bodies, target cells, burr cells, acanthocytes, and thrombocytosis in the peripheral blood (McCarthy *et al.*, 1966; Marsh and Stewart, 1970). Such findings, in the absence of splenectomy, should always raise the suspicion of coeliac disease (Ferguson *et al.*, 1970). Splenic atrophy appears to be part and parcel of a generalized reduction in the lymphoreticular tissues in this disorder. Furthermore, it is not affected by treatment with a gluten-free diet (Trewby *et al.*, 1981) making it more probably the result of constitutional factors in those who are likely to develop coeliac disease and not primarily due to the toxic effects of gluten.

Immunology of coeliac disease

The many immunological disturbances found in coeliac disease have given rise to the belief that this is an immunological disorder. Clinical features lend some support to this concept. The hypersensitivity reaction or gliadin shock, alleviated or prevented by pretreatment with corticosteroids (Krainick *et al.*, 1958) and the improvement in the jejunal mucosa brought about by steroids (Wall *et al.*, 1970) are two such events. The lymphoreticular tissues show fibrotic peripheral lymph nodes (McCarthy *et al.*, 1966) and enlarged and fleshy mesenteric lymph nodes, a possible reaction to antigen from the intestinal tract (Paulley, 1954; Housley *et al.*, 1969). The atrophic spleen may reflect impaired humoral immunity and the increased incidence of auto-immunity found in this disorder (Bullen *et al.*, 1977, 1981). However, it is possible that many of the immunological abnormalities encountered signify nothing more than a response to gluten, and perhaps other antigen, which has crossed a damaged mucosal barrier, so gaining access to the immune system (Hemmings and Williams, 1978; Jackson *et al.*, 1981). There is no evidence as yet that immunological mechanisms initiate mucosal damage, although it is possible that they may perpetuate the lesion. The primary event whereby patients are immunized by gluten is still unexplained, and may well be unrelated to immunological reactions.

Immunologic factors initiating damage to jejunal mucosa

The first point of contact for gluten in the small bowel is with the epithelial cells. Here an abnormality of binding between gluten and the surface of the enterocyte has been suggested as the prime defect in coeliac disease which initiates cell damage (Douglas, 1976; Weiser and Douglas, 1976, 1978). Once the mucosal barrier has been damaged a whole range of disturbances may ensue, perhaps beginning with the production of antigluten antibody. In this regard, the local immune system in the small intestinal mucosa has been implicated as an aetiological factor in coeliac disease (Falchuk and Strober, 1974). In the jejunal mucosa of coeliac patients who are taking a normal diet (Falchuk and Strober, 1972), and in patients who have been on a gluten-free diet followed by a gluten challenge (Loeb *et al.*, 1971), increased IgA and IgM synthesis and antigliadin antibody can be demonstrated (Falchuk and Strober, 1974). Steroids decrease the synthesis of local immunoglobulin in tissue culture (Falchuk and Katz, 1978), and this could be one explanation for their beneficial effects in this disorder (Wall *et al.*, 1970). An increase in IgE-containing cells has been demonstrated in the mucosa of untreated coeliac patients and in many treated with a gluten-free diet. A significant increase in IgE cells can also follow gluten challenge, with evidence of mast cell degranulation and increased eosinophil counts in the post-challenge biopsies (O'Donoghue *et al.*, 1979). Gluten challenge is also associated with an increased tissue concentration of histamine in the mucosa (Challacombe *et al.*, 1980), as well as increased amounts of 5-hydroxytryptamine (Challacombe *et al.*, 1977).

Immune complexes may also be associated with damage to the mucosa, for they have been detected in coeliac disease, together with disturbances of complement (Doe *et al.*, 1973; Mowbray *et al.*, 1973; Teisberg *et al.*, 1977). The morphological abnormalities which are seen (Anand *et al.*, 1981) together with the results from immuno-fluorescence studies, have been interpreted as demonstrating the early deposition of complement and immunoglobulin in the region of the basement membrane. This, and the consumption of complement from serum after gluten challenge, suggests that a local Arthus-type immunological reaction is taking place in the intestinal mucosa (Doe *et al.*, 1974; Shiner and Ballard, 1972, 1973). Of further interest in this respect is the occurrence of soluble antigen–antibody complexes in the serum of some patients after gluten challenge (Doe *et al.*, 1974). The antigen in the complexes has not been identified, but is thought to be gluten or a subfraction (Anand *et al.*, 1981). However, complexes may be innocuous, for they are found in patients with coeliac disease and dermatitis herpetiformis who are symptomless (Mohammed *et al.*, 1976).

Lymphocytes from coeliac patients are sensitized to gluten (Holmes *et al.*, 1976). A subfraction of gluten fraction III markedly stimulated lymphocytes from coeliac patients, as compared with cells from general medical patients and those with other gastrointestinal disorders (Sikora *et al.*, 1976). Using the leucocyte migration inhibition test to investigate cell-mediated immunity against gluten fraction III, the migration indices were significantly lower in treated, but not in untreated, coeliac patients compared with normal control subjects. Overall, about 40 per cent of patients taking a gluten-free diet were below the normal range (Bullen and Losowsky, 1976). Similar results have been found using α-gliadin, such that the test has been regarded by some as specific for coeliac disease (Douwes, 1976; Haeney and Asquith, 1978). Another approach has shown that there may be a population of lymphocytes in the mucosa of coeliac patients which are sensitized to gluten, for it can be shown that when jejunal biopsies from patients taking a normal, but not a gluten-free, diet—or from other non-coeliac individuals—are cultured in the presence of α-gliadin, migration inhibition factor can be demonstrated in the growth medium (Ferguson *et al.*, 1975). Furthermore, coeliac patients may possess a population of lymphocytes directed against their own jejunal mucosa (Scott and Losowsky, 1976).

The question then arises, if cell-mediated reactions are occurring in the small intestinal mucosa in coeliac disease, could these have any role in the formation of the flat biopsy. Atrophy and crypt hyperplasia produced in rats by infection with the parasite *Nippostrongylus brasiliensis* appear to be thymus dependent (Ferguson and Jarrett, 1965). Thymus-dependent mechanisms are also involved in the rejection of grafts of foetal mouse intestine from one strain implanted under the kidney capsule of an adult mouse of another strain, for the number of grafts rejected is considerably reduced when the host mice are thymus-deprived (Ferguson and Parrott, 1973). As rejection proceeds, the villi become shorter and may disappear, while the crypts elongate (MacDonald and Ferguson, 1976). Such changes bear some resemblance to the mucosal abnormalities found in untreated coeliac disease, but there are important differences. Individual enterocytes are well preserved and in about one-quarter of the grafts, intra-epithelial lymphocytes are absent from the mucosa

(MacDonald and Ferguson, 1976). In newly diagnosed coeliac disease an abnormal epithelium infiltrated with lymphocytes is a characteristic finding. Thus while allograft rejection is a useful model, it does not reproduce exactly the abnormalities found in coeliac disease. There are also other difficulties in suggesting that the disorder is due to delayed hypersensitivity. Usually antigen within the mucosa is removed rapidly and it is not clear how gluten could remain in this site long enough for cell-mediated reactions to occur. It is possible that gluten might be held within the mucosa in immune complexes, or in macrophages. A further problem is why the delayed hypersensitivity responses should appear to be localized to the gut. Skin tests with gluten fraction III were macroscopically normal at 48 hours in 21 coeliac patients with one exception (Asquith, 1970), although there were histological changes suggesting that a weak delayed hypersensitivity response can occur in some patients (Asquith, 1974). Subfractions of gluten have been reported to produce positive skin tests, but these are of the Arthus and not the delayed type (Anand and Truelove, 1977; Baker and Read, 1976) and in any case may be found in Crohn's disease and ulcerative colitis.

Immunological disturbances following initial mucosal damage

Whatever the mechanism may be which initiates mucosal damage, with more prolonged exposure to gluten the characteristic jejunal biopsy appearances evolve. These are shortening and disappearance of the villi with damage to the surface cells and elongation of the crypts. The epithelium and lamina propria are increasingly infiltrated by inflammatory cells. Such changes may occur within a few days or weeks but can take months or even years to develop. The processes already discussed above, as possible prime factors in the aetiology of coeliac disease, may well continue to inflict damage on the mucosa. Several mechanisms may be at work simultaneously, and it is clearly not possible to separate initial events from later ones. As the jejunal mucosa becomes permeable to antigens, allowing them access to the circulation, systemic immunological manifestations will occur such as the development of antibodies to food and autoantibodies.

Lymphocytes and plasma cells are found in abnormal numbers in the jejunal mucosa in coeliac disease. Intra-epithelial lymphocyte counts are high in the mucosa of untreated patients and fall to more normal levels following dietary gluten withdrawal (Ferguson and Murray, 1971; Holmes et al., 1974). That gluten within the lumen of the small bowel can influence the lymphocytes is suggested by their wide distribution throughout the epithelium in coeliac patients, rather than being confined to the region below the enterocyte nuclei, as in normal subjects (Ferguson, 1974; Fry et al., 1974). In addition, patients with coeliac disease can be induced to increase the number of intra-epithelial lymphocytes either by a single gluten challenge (Ferguson, 1974; Lancaster-Smith *et al.*, 1975) or by more prolonged gluten feeding (Lancaster-Smith *et al.*, 1975). There are patients with dermatitis herpetiformis, who apparently have normal jejunal biopsies, but with increased lymphocyte counts in the epithelium which fall to normal following dietary gluten withdrawal (Fry *et al.*, 1972). It has thus been considered that lymphocyte infiltration is a manifestation of gluten sensitivity (Fry *et al.*, 1974) and that the earliest change in the epithelium may be invasion by cells sensitized to gluten, adding weight to the immunological hypothesis of coeliac disease.

There are increased numbers of plasma cells and decreased numbers of lymphocytes in the lamina propria of the jejunal mucosa of untreated coeliac patients. Following gluten withdrawal the lymphocyte numbers increase back to normal, and although the plasma cell counts fall, they usually remain elevated (Ferguson *et al.*, 1974; Holmes *et al.*, 1974; Lancaster-Smith *et al.*, 1976a; Montgomery and Shearer, 1974). These changes could be brought about by the local antigenic stimulus of gluten effecting the transformation of lymphocytes to plasma cells in untreated patients. On removal of gluten from the diet the process is reversed, lymphocytes reaccumulate, and plasma cells decrease (Holmes *et al.*, 1974). It is of interest that even where patients show no gross morphological improvement in their jejunal mucosa on a gluten-free diet, they still demonstrate significant improvement in the numbers of plasma cells and lymphocytes (Holmes *et al.*, 1974).

Immunofluorescence has been used to investigate plasma cells in the small intestinal mucosa, and it is generally agreed that IgM cells are increased in children and adults with both treated and untreated coeliac disease (Baklien *et al.*, 1977; Lancaster-Smith *et al.*, 1976b), while IgA cells have been reported as reduced (Douglas *et al.*, 1970), normal (Lancaster-Smith *et al.*, 1974) or increased (Baklien *et al.*, 1977). IgM cells are raised in IgA-deficient individuals, and it has been suggested that in coeliac disease the increased IgM infiltrate is a compensatory mechanism for an impairment in IgA responses (Douglas *et al.*, 1970). *In vitro* studies have shown that the biopsied jejunal mucosa, taken from patients who have been challenged with gluten *in vivo*, responds with an increase in both IgA and IgM (Falchuk and Strober, 1974). With regard to serum immunoglobulins, IgA is elevated (Asquith *et al.*, 1969) and IgM reduced (Hobbs and Hepner, 1968) in the untreated patient. These abnormalities, however, tend to reverse following treatment with a gluten-free diet, suggesting they are of no prime importance. In any event, coeliac disease may develop in IgA-deficient individuals (Mawhinney and Tomkin, 1971; Stokes *et al.*, 1972). IgE levels are usually normal, though raised levels have been reported (Baldo and Wrigley, 1978), but specific allergen tests were negative to many different cereal components.

Antibodies to a variety of foods have been detected in the serum and intestinal juice, not only in coeliac disease, but also in non-coeliac disorders and healthy subjects (Ferguson and Carswell, 1972; Heiner *et al.*, 1962; Taylor *et al.*, 1961). Their presence probably reflects no more than the passage of macromolecules through a damaged intestinal mucosa, and almost certainly they have no role in aetiology. Similarly, anticonnective tissue antibodies probably arise in response to antigens in the food and play no primary part in pathogenesis (Williamson *et al.*, 1976). However, mention should be made of IgA-class reticulin antibodies which appear to be specific for coeliac disease and could be a useful screening test (Magalhaes *et al.*, 1974; Mallas *et al.*, 1977; Eade *et al.*, 1977).

Longer-term problems possibly associated with disturbed immunity

Disturbed immunity in coeliac disease has been considered to predispose to an association with disorders which are also suspected of having an immunological aetiology (Lancaster-Smith *et al.*, 1974; Scott and Losowsky, 1975; Cooper *et al.*, 1978). Several mechanisms may be involved. Thus immune complexes which are found in a large number of disorders may arise from the damaged small intestinal mucosa in coeliac disease and be deposited elsewhere to produce disturbance (Scott and Losowsky, 1975). Support for this concept comes from observations made in dermatitis herpetiformis where immune complexes in the circulation (Mowbray *et al.*, 1973) may play a part in producing the characteristic skin lesions (Seah *et al.*, 1973). Organ-specific autoimmune endocrinopathies and some other autoimmune diseases may result from abnormal immune surveillance (Volpe, 1977) which may also be relevant in coeliac disease (MacLaurin *et al.*, 1971). It is generally considered that subjects with the HLA B8 antigen are predisposed to develop immunological disturbance, and this antigen is present in the majority of coeliac patients (Stokes *et al.*, 1972). The passage of toxic substances and antigens across the damaged small intestinal mucosa and the presence of various autoantibodies (Hodgson *et al.*, 1976) may also play a part in the development of associated immunological disturbance. Finally, selective IgA deficiency appears to predispose to atopy (Collin-Williams *et al.*, 1971) and it has been suggested that atopy in coeliac disease may be due to abnormal mucosal IgA responses (Hodgson *et al.*, 1976). The commonest associations are diabetes mellitus, pulmonary disorders, liver disease, and thyroid problems. It is important that these second diagnoses should not be overlooked.

Lastly, disturbed immunity may possibly play a part in the development of the most serious complication of coeliac disease, namely lymphoma (Holmes *et al.*, 1976). Mechanisms suggested have included lymphoid hyperactivity in the jejunal mucosa (Austad *et al.*, 1967) and it has also been proposed that they may depend on the HLA profile of coeliac patients (Stokes *et al.*, 1972) and reduced immune surveillance (MacLaurin *et al.*, 1971).

A summary of the present position regarding the aetiology of coeliac disease may be attempted at this point. The 'missing peptidase' hypothesis has become virtually untenable (Sterchi and Woodley, 1978), although it still commands some support (Cornell and Rolles, 1978). There is strong evidence that constitutional factors play an important and probably essential role in the development of the condition (Pena et al., 1978). Given the constitutional background, then a number of influences acting together or separately, such as infection, other stresses or the early presentation of gluten to the immature intestine, may trigger the mechanism which initiates mucosal damage. Undoubtedly, the binding of gluten to the surface of the enterocytes and subsequent immunological reactions are of importance in the evolution of the mucosal changes so characteristic of coeliac disease. There is still no knowledge of the identity of the specific toxic substance in gluten, whether it is a pure peptide, which seems unlikely, a glycoprotein, or some other antigen. There remains an immense unexplored field of great technical complexity which may provide the answer. Finally, the crucial question remains why only a few people in the population develop coeliac disease although all are exposed to gluten.

Intolerance to milk, soy protein, eggs, and other foods and non-coeliac gluten intolerance

There is increasing evidence that in susceptible individuals certain foods may cause clinical disorder, and that patients with coeliac disease resulting from gluten intolerance may be only part of a larger group in whom other antigens may be capable of setting in motion events leading to varying degrees of damage to the jejunal mucosa. In this regard intolerance to milk, eggs, soy protein and other foods, and non-coeliac gluten intolerance require consideration.

Milk

In coeliac disease there is usually some degree of lactose intolerance depending, it is presumed, on the severity of the mucosal damage. In most patients, however, this intolerance is removed on exclusion of gluten from the diet except for those with a constitutional alactasia, necessitating a lactose- and gluten-free diet. There is an additional cause of milk intolerance in that patients may be upset by milk protein, a defect which has been particularly studied in infancy and childhood. Its mechanism is not known. Whether milk protein can adversely affect the jejunal mucosa in adults is uncertain. In one of our adult patients, restoration of normal histology did not take place until both milk and gluten were excluded from the diet.

Cow's milk protein intolerance occurs in infants and usually is a temporary condition, clearing before the age of 2 years. It is associated with similar symptoms to those of gluten intolerance, for example diarrhoea, vomiting, failure to thrive, steatorrhoea, and a jejunal mucosa similar to that found in untreated coeliac disease, though in general not so severe (Visakorpi, 1979). Similar immunological features, such as a raised level of IgA in the serum and alterations in the number of immunoglobulin-producing cells in the jejunal mucosa, are also present. The abnormalities resolve on removal of milk from the diet. Furthermore, though the jejunal mucosal damage is apparently identical to that seen in coeliac disease, it returns to normal on removal of milk from the diet despite continuing gluten ingestion (Kuitenen et al., 1975). Of further interest is that, while the majority of patients also have transient gluten intolerance, about 10 per cent eventually develop coeliac disease. The similarity of the changes produced in the intestinal mucosa to those in coeliac disease has led to the suggestion that the mechanism is also similar (Visakorpi, 1979). However, some protection appears to be given by sodium cromoglycate (Freier and Berger, 1973), which does not apply in coeliac disease.

Eggs

Eggs are one of the common allergens recognized as causing asthma and eczema. They can also cause problems in coeliac disease and three of our patients did not regain normal health until both eggs and gluten had been excluded from their diet. Two interesting case reports illustrate some of the problems—the one illustrating the diagnostic difficulties and the other strongly suggesting that eggs may be responsible for damage to the intestinal mucosa. It had been noted that coeliac disease was associated with diffuse interstitial lung disease and that this disorder, particularly since it was associated with serum antibodies against avian-derived antigens, was possibly an autoimmune fibrosing alveolitis. Furthermore, when the patients were removed from contact with birds, the lung condition improved or did not deteriorate, suggesting that the pulmonary condition was bird-fancier's lung. A survey of 15 of these patients (Berrill et al., 1975) was carried out, and of the nine selected for jejunal biopsy, five had flat specimens. The significance of these avian antigens is uncertain, for they may occur in coeliac patients who have no evidence of lung disease or of contact with birds and are not the ones associated with bird-fancier's lung (Faux et al., 1978; Hendrick et al., 1978). The antigen in coeliac disease was found to reside is hen egg yolk. Of the five patients reported by Berrill et al. (1975) four responded to a gluten-free diet, but the fifth who had previously been reported by Hood and Mason (1970, case 2), responded only to a poultry-free diet. We are indebted to Dr Margot Shiner for further details concerning this patient. Treatment with various exclusion diets over 3–4 years including gluten, eggs, poultry, and milk has not brought about any improvement in her jejunal biopsy. Diarrhoea and abdominal pain follows 3–6 hours after the ingestion of chicken, turkey, or eggs. At present, she maintains good health on a gluten-containing diet, but with chicken and eggs excluded. Of interest was the markedly increased immunofluorescent staining of IgE-containing cells in the jejunal mucosa. The serum levels for IgE were normal. IgE-specific antibodies (RAST) were negative for egg white; milk; fish; cat, dog, and horse hairs; house-dust mites; wheat; and timothy grass pollen.

An equally important case report (Baker and Rosenberg, 1978) concerns a 44-year-old woman who presented with diarrhoea and severe weight loss: the jejunal biopsy findings were compatible with coeliac disease. However, she failed to make a satisfactory response to a gluten-free diet and was diagnosed as having refractory sprue by the centre that had introduced that term. Subsequent investigation elsewhere showed clearly that vomiting, severe diarrhoea, and hypotension followed the ingestion of egg, chicken, or tuna fish within 2 hours. Elimination of these foods, while still on a gluten-free diet, led to restoration of normal villi. Unfortunately, she refuses gluten challenge. She takes milk and milk proteins without difficulty. Though the reactions were associated with marked leucocytosis, there was no eosinophilia in the blood.

Soy protein

Soy protein has been used in the treatment of coeliac disease as a replacement for gluten and also as a substitute for milk protein in cow's milk intolerance. However, it is now clear from a number of reports that soy protein itself may produce changes in the small intestinal mucosa 'identical with those encountered in coeliac disease' (Ament and Rubin, 1972); though it must be pointed out that microulceration, polymorphonuclear infiltration, oedema, and haemorrhage are not findings usually seen in the jejunal mucosa in coeliac disease. The clinical symptoms are vomiting, diarrhoea, shock, fever, and asthma. The reaction is reversible on withdrawal of soy protein and is not associated with consumption of complement, blood eosinophilia, or eosinophilic infiltration of the jejunal mucosa. Some protection is afforded by sodium cromoglycate (Kocoshis and Gryboski, 1979).

Eosinophilic gastroenteritis is a relatively uncommon disorder (Klein *et al.*, 1970; Leinbach and Rubin, 1970), characterized by gastrointestinal symptoms following the ingestion of a specific food, eosinophilia, and an eosinophilic cellular infiltrate of some part of the intestinal tract. Complete loss of villi may occur in some patients, though patchy in distribution. Diarrhoea, abdominal pain and vomiting have occurred after soy protein and steak, but without any clear-cut reaction either in the eosinophils of the peripheral blood or of the eosinophilic infiltration of the jejunal mucosa. Elimination diets have produced dramatic clinical improvement but eventually the symptoms return. It was concluded that eosinophilic gastroenteritis is not a simple reversible allergic reaction to specific foods but rather a self-perpetuating process aggravated periodically by various food antigens. In some the process required control by corticosteroid therapy. The effect of sodium cromoglycate does not appear to have been tried.

Non-coeliac gluten intolerance

In non-coeliac patients with food allergy or intolerance, the common symptoms are asthma, eczema, urticaria, angioedema, abdominal pain, vomiting, or diarrhoea, either appearing immediately or delayed for 2 hours. The commonest food allergens causing problems in non-coeliacs are those in milk, eggs, fish, and nuts but it is of considerable interest that cereals — wheat, rye, barley, and oats — are the offending articles in a minority of non-coeliac patients with asthma and eczema. The value of skin tests and allergen-specific tests (RAST) in detecting such patients is limited (Aas, 1978), particularly in those with a non-immediate response — for the tests are more likely to be negative than positive (Wraith et al., 1979). Whether any of these patients have coeliac disease or show any reaction in their jejunal mucosa is doubtful, but jejunal biopsies have rarely been carried out. Pock-Steen (1973) discussed the role of gluten in chronic or intermittent dyspepsia in non-coeliac subjects, but undoubtedly included a number of coeliac patients (jejunal mucosa abnormalities just short of a flat biopsy, steatorrhoea after gluten challenge, and two patients with dermatitis herpetiformis). The occasional coeliac patient will show a dramatic recovery from eczema on a gluten-free diet (Friedman and Hare, 1965). On the other hand RAST studies in coeliac disease using a variety of cereal antigens including α-gliadin have been negative, even when the serum IgE levels were increased (Baldo and Wrigley, 1978).

The use of sodium cromoglycate in food allergy has had some success in protecting patients against asthma and eczema following the oral administration of antigens (Bleumink, 1979). The fact that it can also protect some patients with chronic diarrhoea, in whom coeliac disease, soy protein, and cow's milk intolerance had been excluded, suggests that there are a number of foods which can cause gastrointestinal symptoms only (Bolin, 1980). It is not really surprising then, with the increasing interest in food allergens, that patients are encountered who are intolerant of gluten but who otherwise show none of the characteristics of coeliac disease (Dahl, 1979; Jonas, 1978).

Nine such patients have been carefully studied, all women and of English stock and with an absence of atopic disease personally or in their relatives (Cooper et al., 1980b). All had suffered with persistent diarrhoea for periods up to 20 years, averaging 5 years, which was often socially incapacitating and nocturnal. Defaecation tended to be explosive with watery, offensive stools though without steatorrhoea. Central abdominal pain was common, as was abdominal distension, malaise, and lassitude. The majority had lost weight of up to 9.5 kg. Three had recurrent aphthous stomatitis. Investigations showed haemoglobins varying from 13.1 g/dl to 14.7 g/dl, with normal white cell counts and no eosinophilia. Serum levels of albumin, globulin, calcium, and alkaline phosphatase were normal. Multiple jejunal biopsies, on at least two separate occasions, were all macroscopically normal. There were, however, significant increases in the plasma cells of the lamina propria and lymphocytes in the epithelial cell layer, though significantly less than the counts found in untreated coeliac disease. Eosinophilic cellular infiltration was absent. The brush-border enzymes, lactase, and maltase were within normal limits. The response of these patients to a gluten-free diet was dramatic, for within 2 weeks a sense of well-being had returned, the stool frequency had fallen to 1 to 2 per day, and abdominal distension and pain and aphthous stomatitis had disappeared. Repeat jejunal biopsies showed a return to normal levels of the cellular infiltration. Repeated gluten challenges caused a recurrence of symptoms within 3–4 hours. These symptoms sometimes lasted as long as a week and included diarrhoea, malaise, headache, swollen lips, and abdominal pain. Twenty-four hours after challenge there was an increase in the plasma cells of the lamina propria but not of the epithelial lymphocytes. There was no increased eosinophilic infiltrate. The serum, before and 24 hours after challenge, showed no change in the normal levels of complement C1q, C3, C4, C6, and C7, nor were antigluten antibodies found at any time. IgG and IgA antireticulin antibodies were not detected either in the serum or in the jejunal juice. Neither the serum IgE levels nor blood eosinophil numbers showed any change at 24 hours after challenge, but remained within normal limits. A further patient we have seen with this condition was not benefited by sodium cromoglycate. Thus immunological disturbances were not found in these patients, apart from minor but significant changes in plasma cell and lymphocyte counts in the jejunal mucosa. There was no evidence of type I (atopic) hypersensitivity, such as an eosinophilia or raised serum levels of IgE, or of allergic gastroenteropathy (absence of mucosal eosinophilic infiltrate). Normal levels of serum albumin did not support a protein-losing enteropathy. The absence of change in complement levels and of detectable breakdown products after gluten challenge make a type II (cytotoxic) or type III (immune complex) immune reaction unlikely, as does the lack of gluten antibodies. The occurrence of abdominal symptoms within 12 hours is perhaps a little early for a type IV cell-mediated hypersensitivity reaction, and the jejunal mucosa did not show the characteristic changes. The mechanism is completely unknown. It could be comparable to the mechanism encountered in cholera, when watery diarrhoea results from the induction of adenyl cyclase activity by the surface-bound enterotoxin without producing significant mucosal change (Sharpe and Hynie, 1971); and it is possible that some component of gluten could be acting as a lectin. The mucosal defect promoting the abnormal binding of gluten could have been uncovered by an event such as an infection.

The observations made by Anderson et al. (1981) are also of some importance, and offer another possible explanation for food intolerance. They pointed out that whilst lactose was often responsible for flatulence, abdominal discomfort, and diarrhoea, it was also possible that sucrose or starch might have similar effects. Using breath hydrogen methods, they demonstrated that virtually all normal subjects failed to absorb the carbohydrate of white all-purpose flour completely. They noted that this malabsorption of starch was corrected on a gluten-free diet and furthermore, and surprisingly, was not reproduced when gluten was added to the gluten-free diet. Sucrose and rice flour appeared to be absorbed completely. Since the flour of all-purpose wheat comprises granules with a starch core surrounded by a protein network, they suggested that the explanation of their findings lay in the damage caused to these granules when extracting gluten and that the malabsorption of starch from the untreated flour was in some way due to the interaction of the starch and protein moieties of the wheat flour.

This cause for malabsorption may be the explanation of the beneficial effect of a gluten-free diet noted in tropical sprue. One such report did not exclude the possibility of coeliac disease as an explanation (Cancio et al., 1961). However, 10 Puerto Rican patients treated for 3–10 weeks on a gluten-free diet showed a clinical remission in four and histological improvement of their jejunal biopsies in five. Gluten feeding to 11 patients in remission, including two already on a gluten-free diet, produced steatorrhoea in seven and mild mucosal changes (Bayless and Swanson, 1964).

There is now good evidence that a proportion of those suffering from moderately severe, recurrent aphthous stomatitis, unassociated with any other disease, may obtain complete remission on a gluten-free diet. Three of our patients with non-coeliac diarrhoea with such symptoms have experienced complete remission for the past 5 years (Cooper et al., 1980). Wray (1981) reported that five amongst 20 patients with recurrent stomatitis obtained similar remission. He noted that basophils from some of these patients with normal jejunal biopsies released histamine on incubation with a variety of foods including cereals and wheat. The possibility of immunological factors playing some part is suggested by the significantly increased number of plasma cells found in the lamina propria of the non-coeliac patients with recurrent aphthous ulceration, indicating reaction to an antigen from the gut (Ferguson et al., 1976). One of these patients subsequently treated with a gluten-free diet obtained complete remission of her symptoms. The possible beneficial effect of exclusion of other foods has not been reported.

Inflammatory bowel disease

Ulcerative colitis

The idea that ulcerative colitis was an allergic disorder was put forward more than 50 years ago. Milk was thought to be involved in 84 per cent of cases and to be the direct aetiological cause in 40 per cent (Andresen, 1942). This suggestion received some support from Truelove (1961) who found that 13 amongst 200 patients experienced a remission when milk was withdrawn, and relapsed when milk was reintroduced.

An immunological cause for the disorder was suspected from the findings of an increased incidence of antibodies against milk proteins in patients compared with controls (Taylor and Truelove, 1961; Wright and Truelove, 1965b). However, this observation was not confirmed (Sewell et al., 1963; Dudek et al., 1965; Jewell and Truelove, 1972) and hypolactasia was thought to be the cause of increased symptoms following milk ingestion (Binder et al., 1964; Pena and Truelove, 1973). However, reactions to milk ingestion suggestive of an allergic reaction do occur. A condition like ulcerative colitis has been described in infancy following milk (Gryboski et al., 1966), while in one of our adult patients a severe reaction occurred within 3 hours of taking milk, with marked pyrexia, tachycardia, hypotension, and frequent bowel actions. Other features of an allergic reaction may be found, such as increased numbers of eosinophils in the blood and mucosa (Wright and Truelove, 1966; Buckell et al., 1978), although there is no increase in IgE-containing immunocytes in the rectal mucosa (Lloyd et al., 1975). Serum IgE levels are normal while allergen-specific tests (RAST) to egg white, milk, wheat, rye, oats, fish, and peanuts were negative in one series (Jones et al., 1981). The results of therapy with sodium cromoglycate have been varied, with some reporting improvement (Heatley et al., 1975; Mani et al., 1976) while others report no benefit (Buckell et al., 1978; Dronfield and Langman, 1978). A defect of all the trials was the relative inactivity of the disease at the time of the study, and in some the concomitant administration of salazopyrine and steroids. The possible benefit in subgroups is difficult to exclude.

Attempts to implicate other foods in ulcerative colitis have given negative results. A gluten-free diet was ineffective in one series (Wright and Truelove, 1965a). However, rectal bleeding and diarrhoea similar to that following milk in infants has occurred with soy protein (Ament and Rubin, 1972).

Crohn's disease

The role of diet as a factor in the aetiology of Crohn's disease has been considered as a possible explanation for the increased incidence of this condition noted in recent years, coinciding with the greater consumption of processed foods and food additives. It has been suggested that there is a highly significant correlation between eating cornflakes and the development of Crohn's disease (James, 1977) although this has been denied (Archer and Harvey, 1978; Rawcliffe and Truelove, 1978). More refined sugar and less fibre in the diet has also been regarded as important in this context (Silkoff et al., 1980; Thornton et al., 1979). Milk, as in ulcerative colitis, is responsible for abdominal discomfort and persistent diarrhoea in an appreciable number of patients, and is associated with a reduction in the disaccharidase activity of the jejunal mucosa (Chalfin and Holt, 1967; Dunne *et al.*, 1977). It must be admitted that there is no evidence to suggest that any of these foods are a primary cause of Crohn's disease.

Little has been published on the effect of sodium cromoglycate in Crohn's disease although benefit has been claimed in an isolated case report (Henderson and Hishon, 1978). Favourable results have also been reported for a gluten-free diet (Rudman *et al.*, 1971). We have used this diet occasionally but obtained no improvement in two patients with diffuse jejunoileitis. Some improvement in the feeling of well-being and in the skin lesions and bowel symptoms was achieved in two patients who also had dermatitis herpetiformis (with normal jejunal biopsies and IgA deposits in the skin). The significance of this is difficult to interpret, since a gluten-free diet is always liable to produce some symptomatic improvement by a non-specific effect in the reduction of flatulence, distension, and flatus.

Elemental diets in seven patients with diffuse jejunoileitis decreased the gastrointestinal protein loss and improved the serum albumin levels (Logan *et al.*, 1981). Such diets are virtually free from dietary allergens which, it was suggested, might explain their value. There was however no indication of the zinc and magnesium status of the patients or their intake in the diet. Both these elements are important in the protein metabolism of severely malnourished patients with Crohn's disease. The important point was however made, that suitable dietary manipulations could be highly beneficial in Crohn's disease.

Our own policy in the long-term supervision of more than 500 patients with this disorder has been to advise them to eat foods they like and avoid those that dislike *them*; with the additional admonition to monitor carefully the effects of milk and milk products, and to take care with cabbage stalks, cauliflower stalks, pieces of orange, and other fibrous fruits which are liable to cause abdominal colic. Milk, cheese, eggs, and tomatoes are the common foods which cause patients problems.

REFERENCES

Aas, K. (1978). The diagnosis of hypersensitivity to ingested foods. Reliability of skin prick testing and the radioallergosorbent test with different materials. *Clinical Allergy*, **8**, 39–50.

Ament, M. E., and Rubin, C. E. (1972). Soy protein. Another cause of the flat lesion. *Gastroenterology*, **62**, 227–34.

Anand, B. S., Piris, J., Jerrome, D. W., Offord, R. E., and Truelove, S. C. (1981). The timing of histological damage following a single challenge with gluten in treated coeliac disease. *Quarterly Journal of Medicine*, **50**, 83–93.

Anand, B. S., and Truelove, S. C. (1977). Skin test for coeliac disease using a subfraction of gluten. *Lancet*, **1**, 118–20.

Andersen, D. H. (1947). Coeliac syndrome: relationship of coeliac disease, starch intolerance and steatorrhoea. *Journal of Paediatrics*, **30**, 564–82.

Anderson, I. H., Levine, A. S., and Levitt, M. D. (1981). Incomplete absorption of the carbohydrate in all-purpose flour. *New England Journal of Medicine*, **304**, 891–2.

Andresen, A. F. R. (1942). Ulcerative colitis—an allergic phenomenon. *American Journal of Digestive Disease*, **9**, 91–8.

Archer, L. N. J., and Harvey, R. F. (1978). Breakfast and Crohn's disease—II. *British Medical Journal*, **3**, 540.

Ashkenazi, A., Krasilowsky, D., Levin, S., Idar, D., Kalian, M., Or, A., Ginat, Y., and Halperin, B. (1979). Immunologic reaction of psychotic patients to fractions of gluten. *American Journal of Psychotherapy*, **10**, 1306–9.

Asquith, P. (1970). Adult coeliac disease. A clinical, morphological and immunological study. MD thesis, Birmingham University.

Asquith, P. (1974). Immunology. *Clinics in Gastroenterology*, **3**, 213–34.

Asquith, P., Thompson, R. A., and Cooke, W. T. (1969). Serum immunoglobulins in adult coeliac disease. *Lancet*, **2**, 129–31.

Austad, W. I., Cornes, J. S., Gough, K. R., McCarthy, C. F., and Read, A. E. (1967). Steatorrhoea and malignant lymphoma. The relationship of malignant tumours of lymphoid tissue and coeliac disease. *American Journal of Digestive Disease*, **12**, 475–90.

Baker, A. L., and Rosenberg, I. H. (1978). Refractory sprue: recovery after removal of non-gluten dietary proteins. *Annals of Internal Medicine*, **89**, 505–8.

Baker, P. G., and Read, A. E. (1976). Positive skin reactions to gluten in coeliac disease. *Quarterly Journal of Medicine*, **45**, 603–10.

Baklien, K., Brandtzaeg, P., and Fausa, O. (1977). Immunoglobulins in jejunal mucosa and serum in patients with adult coeliac disease. *Scandinavian Journal of Gastroenterology*, **12**, 149–59.

Baldo, B. A., and Wrigley, C. W. (1978). IgE antibodies to wheat flour components. Studies with sera from subjects with baker's asthma or coeliac condition. *Clinical Allergy*, **8**, 109–24.

Bayless, T. M., and Swanson, V. L. (1964). Comparison of tropical sprue and adult coeliac disease (non-tropical sprue). *Gastroenterology*, **46**, 731.

Benn, A., and Cooke, W. T. (1971). Intraluminal pH of duodenum and jejunum in fasting subjects with normal and abnormal gastric or pancreatic function. *Scandinavian Journal of Gastroenterology*, **6**, 313–17.

Berrill, W. T., Eade, O. E., Fitzpatrick, P. F., Hyde, I., MacLeod, W. M., and Wright, R. (1975). Bird fancier's lung and jejunal villous atrophy. *Lancet*, **2**, 1006–8.

Binder, H. J., Gryboski, J. D., Thayer, W. R., and Spiro, H. M. (1964). Intolerance to milk in ulcerative colitis. *American Journal of Digestive Disease*, **11**, 858–64.

Blainey, J. D., Cooke, W. T., Quinton, A., and Scott, K. W. (1954). The measurement of total exchangeable potassium in man with particular reference to patients with steatorrhoea. *Clinical Science*, **13**, 165–76.

Blair, J. A., and Matty, A. J. (1974). Acid microclimate in intestinal absorption. *Clinics in Gastroenterology*, **3**, 183–97.

Bleumink, E. (1979). Food allergy and the gastrointestinal tract. In: *Immunology of the Gastrointestinal Tract* (ed. P. Asquith). Churchill-Livingstone, Edinburgh, pp.195–213.

Bolin, T. D. (1980). Use of oral sodium cromoglycate in persistent diarrhoea. *Gut*, **21**, 848–50.

Buckell, N. A., Gould, S. R., Day, D. W., Lennard-Jones, J. E., and Edwards, A. M. (1978). Controlled trial of sodium cromoglycate in chronic persistent ulcerative colitis. *Gut*, **19**, 1140–3.

Bullen, A. W., Hall, R., Gowland, G., and Losowsky, M. S. (1977). Immunity and the hyposplenism of coeliac disease. *Gut*, **18**, 961-2.

Bullen, A. W., Hall, R., Gowland, G., Rajah, S., and Losowsky, M. S. (1981). Hyposplenism, adult coeliac disease and autoimmunity. *Gut*, **22**, 28-33.

Bullen, A. W., and Losowsky, M. S. (1976). Cell mediated immunity to gluten fraction III in adult coeliac disease. *Gut*, **17**, 813.

Cancio, M., Rodriques-Molina, R., and Asenho, C. F. (1961). Gluten and tropical sprue. *American Journal of Tropical Medicine and Hygiene*, **10**, 783-9.

Carter, C., Sheldon, W., and Walker, C. (1959). The inheritance of coeliac disease. *Annals of Human Genetics*, **23**, 266-78.

Chalfin, D., and Holt, P. R. (1967). Lactase deficiency in ulcerative colitis, regional enteritis and viral hepatitis. *American Journal of Digestive Disease*, **12**, 81-7.

Challacombe, D. N., Dawkins, P. D., and Baker, P. (1977). Increased tissue concentrations of 5-hydroxytryptamine in duodenal mucosa of patients with coeliac disease. *Gut*, **18**, 882-6.

Challacombe, D. N., Edwards, J. P., and Baylis, J. M. (1980). Histamine release in post challenge coeliac disease. *Lancet*, **1**, 202.

Ciclitira, P. J., Hunter, J. O., and Lennox, E. S. (1980). Clinical testing of bread made from nullisomic 6A wheats in coeliac patients. *Lancet*, **2**, 234-5.

Collin-Williams, C., Chiu, A. W., and Varga, E. A. (1971). The relationship of atopic disease and immunoglobulin levels with special reference to selective IgA deficiency. *Clinical Allergy*, **1**, 381-6.

Cooke, W. T. (1957). Water and electrolyte upsets in the steatorrhoea syndrome. *Journal of the Mount Sinai Hospital*, **24**, 221-31.

Cooke, W. T. (1976). Neurologic manifestations of malabsorption. In: *Handbook of Clinical Neurology* (ed. H. L. Klawans). North Holland Publishing Company, Amsterdam, **28**, 225-41.

Cooke, W. T., and Holmes, G. K. T. (1977). Non-responsive coeliac disease. *British Medical Journal*, **2**, 1415.

Cooke, W. T., Johnson, A. G., and Wolff, A. L. (1966). Vital staining and electron microscopy of the intramuscular nerve endings in the neuropathy of adult coeliac disease. *Brain*, **89**, 663-82.

Cooke, W. T., and Smith, W. T. (1966). Neurological disorders associated with adult coeliac disease. *Brain*, **89**, 683-722.

Cooke, W. T., Thomas, G., Mangall, D., and Cross, H. (1953). Observations of the faecal extraction of total solids, nitrogen, sodium, potassium, water and fat in the steatorrhoea syndrome. *Clinical Science*, **12**, 223-34.

Cooper, B. T., Holmes, G. K. T., and Cooke, W. T. (1978). Coeliac disease and immunological disorders. *British Medical Journal*, **1**, 537-9.

Cooper, B. T., Holmes, G. K. T., Ferguson, R., and Cooke, W. T. (1980a). Coeliac disease and malignancy. *Medicine (Baltimore)*, **59**, 249-61.

Cooper, B. T., Holmes, G. K. T., Ferguson, R., Thompson, R. A., Allan, R. N., and Cooke, W. T. (1980b). Gluten-sensitive diarrhoea without evidence of coeliac disease. *Gastroenterology*, **79**, 801-6.

Cornell, H. J., and Rolles, C. J. (1978). Further evidence of a primary mucosal defect in coeliac disease. *Gut*, **19**, 253-9.

Dahl, R. (1979). Wheat sensitive—but not coeliac. *Lancet*, **1**, 44-5.

Davidson, G. P., and Townley, R. R. W. (1977). Structural and functional abnormalities of the small intestine due to nutritional folic acid deficiency in infancy. *Journal of Paediatrics*, **90**, 590-4.

Davidson, L. S. P., and Fountain, J. R. (1950). Incidence of the sprue syndrome with some observations on the natural history. *British Medical Journal*, **1**, 1157-61.

Dicke, W. K. (1950). Coeliakie een onderzok naar de nadelige invloed van sommige graansoorten op de lijder aan coeliakie. Doctoral Thesis, University of Utrecht, Netherlands.

Doe, W. F., Booth, C. C., and Brown, D. L. (1973). Evidence for complement binding immune complexes in adult coeliac disease, Crohn's disease and ulcerative colitis. *Lancet*, **1**, 402–3.

Doe, W. F., Henry, K., and Booth, C. C. (1974). Complement in coeliac disease. In: *Coeliac Disease* (eds W. T. J. M. Hekkens, and A. S. Pena). Stenfert Kroese, Leiden, pp.189–96.

Dohan, F. C. (1966). Cereals and schizophrenia: data and hypothesis. *Acta Psychiatrica Scandinavica*, **42**, 125–52.

Dohan, F. C., and Glasberger, J. C. (1973). Relapsed schizophrenics: earlier discharge from hospital after cereal-free milk-free diet. *American Journal of Psychiatry*, **130**, 685–8.

Doherty, M., and Barry, R. E. (1981). Gluten induced mucosal changes in subjects without overt small bowel disease. *Lancet*, **1**, 517–20.

Douglas, A. P. (1976). The binding of a glycopeptide component of wheat gluten to intestinal mucosa of normal and coeliac human subjects. *Clinica Chimica Acta*, **73**, 357–61.

Douglas, A. P., Crabbe, P. A., and Hobbs, J. R. (1970). Immunochemical studies of the serum, intestinal secretions and intestinal mucosa in patients with adult coeliac disease and other forms of coeliac syndrome. *Gastroenterology*, **59**, 414–25.

Douwes, F. R. (1976). Gluten and lymphocyte sensitisation in coeliac disease. *Lancet*, **2**, 1353.

Dronfield, M. W., and Langman, M. J. S. (1978). Comparative trial of sulphasalazine and oral sodium cromoglycate in the maintenance of remission in ulcerative colitis. *Gut*, **19**, 1136–9.

Dudek, B., Spiro, H. M., and Thayer, W. R. (1965). A study of ulcerative colitis and circulating antibodies to milk protein. *Gastroenterology*, **49**, 544–7.

Dunne, W. T., Cooke, W. T., and Allan, R. N. (1977). Enzymatic and morphometric evidence for Crohn's disease as a diffuse lesion of the gastrointestinal tract. *Gut*, **18**, 290–4.

Eade, O. E., Lloyd, R. S., Lang, C., and Wright, R. (1977). IgA and IgG reticulin antibodies in coeliac and non-coeliac patients. *Gut*, **18**, 991–3.

Egan-Mitchell, B., Fottrell, P. F., and McNicholl, B. (1981). Early or pre-coeliac mucosa: development of gluten enteropathy. *Gut*, **22**, 65–9.

Ewart, J. A. D. (1970). Chemistry of wheat proteins. In: *Coeliac Disease* (eds C. C. Booth, and R. H. Dowling). Churchill-Livingstone, Edinburgh, pp.1–9.

Falchuk, Z. M., and Katz, A. J. (1978). Organ culture model of gluten-sensitive enteropathy. In: *Perspectives in Coeliac Disease* (eds B. McNicholl, C. F. McCarthy, and P. F. Fottrell). MTP Press, Lancaster, pp.65–72.

Falchuk, Z. M., and Strober, W. (1972). Increased jejunal immunoglobulin synthesis in patients with non-tropical sprue as measured by a solid phase immunoadsorption technique. *Journal of Laboratory and Clinical Medicine*, **79**, 1004–13.

Falchuk, Z. M., and Strober, W. (1974). Gluten sensitive enteropathy: synthesis of antigliadin antibody in vitro. *Gut*, **15**, 947–52.

Faux, A., Hendrick, D. J., and Anand, B. S. (1978). Precipitins to different avian serum antigens in bird fancier's lung and coeliac disease. *Clinical Allergy*, **8**, 101–8.

Ferguson, A. (1974). Lymphocytes in coeliac disease. In: *Coeliac Disease* (eds W. T. J. M. Hekkens, and A. S. Pena). Stenfert Kroese, Leiden, pp.265–276.

Ferguson, A., and Carswell, F. (1972). Precipitins to dietary proteins in serum and upper intestinal secretions of coeliac children. *British Medical Journal*, **1**, 75–7.

Ferguson, A., Hutton, M. M., Maxwell, J. D., and Murray, D. (1970). Adult coeliac disease in hyposplenic patients. *Lancet*, **1**, 163–4.

Ferguson, A., and Jarrett, E. E. E. (1965). Hypersensitivity reactions in the small intestine. I. Thymus dependence of experimental partial villous atrophy. *Gut*, **16**, 114–17.

Ferguson, A., McClure, J. P., MacDonald, T. T., and Holden, R. J. (1975). Cell mediated immunity to gliadin within the small intestinal mucosa in coeliac disease. *Lancet*, **1**, 895–7.

Ferguson, A., and Murray, D. (1971). Quantitation of intraepithelial lymphocytes in human jejunum. *Gut*, **12**, 988–94.

Ferguson, A., and Parrott, D. M. V. (1973). Histopathology and time course of rejection of allografts of mouse small intestine. *Transplantation*, **15**, 546–54.

Ferguson, R., Asquith, P., and Cooke, W. T. (1974). The jejunal cellular infiltrate in coeliac disease complicated by lymphoma. *Gut*, **15**, 458–61.

Ferguson, R., Basu, M. K., Asquith, P., and Cooke, W. T. (1976). Jejunal mucosal abnormalities in patients with recurrent aphthous ulceration. *British Medical Journal*, **1**, 11–13.

Ferguson, R., Holmes, G. K. T., and Cooke, W. T. (1982). Coeliac disease, fertility and pregnancy. *Scandinavian Journal of Gastroenterology*, **17**, 65–8.

Fordtran, J. S., Rector, F. C., Locklear, T. W., and Ewton, M. F. (1967). Water and solute movement in the small intestine of patients with sprue. *Journal of Clinical Investigation*, **46**, 287–98.

Freier, S., and Berger, H. (1973). Disodium cromoglycate in gastrointestinal protein intolerance. *Lancet*, **1**, 913–15.

Friedman, M., and Hare, P. J. (1965). Gluten sensitive enteropathy and eczema. *Lancet*, **1**, 521–4.

Fry, L., Seah, P. P., Harper, P. G., Hoffbrand, A. V., and McMinn, R. M. H. (1974). The small intestine in dermatitis herpetiformis. *Journal of Clinical Pathology*, **27**, 817–24.

Fry, L., Seah, P. P., McMinn, R. M. H., and Hoffrand, A. V. (1972). Lymphocytic infiltration of epithelium in diagnosis of gluten sensitive enteropathy. *British Medical Journal*, **3**, 371–4.

Fry, L., Swain, F., Leonard, J., and McMinn, R. M. H. (1981). Disodium cromoglycate in dermatitis herpetiformis. *British Journal of Dermatology*, **105**, 83–6.

Gee, S. (1888). On the coeliac affection. *St. Bartholomew's Hospital Reports*, **24**, 17–20.

Groll, A., Candy, D. C. A., Preece, M. A., Tanner, J. M., and Harries, J. T. (1980). Short stature as the primary manifestation of coeliac disease. *Lancet*, **2**, 1097–9.

Gryboski, J. D., Burkle, F., and Hillman, R. (1966). Milk induced colitis in an infant. *Paediatrics*, **38**, 299–302.

Haeney, M. R., and Asquith, P. (1978). Inhibition of leucocyte migration by α-gliadin in patients with gastrointestinal disease: its specificity with respect to α-gliadin and coeliac disease. In: *Perspectives in Coeliac Disease* (eds B. McNicholl, C. F. McCarthy, and P. F. Fottrell). MTP Press, Lancaster, pp.229–42.

Harris, O. D., Cooke, W. T., Thompson, H., and Waterhouse, J. A. H. (1967). Malignancy in adult coeliac disease and idiopathic steatorrhoea. *American Journal of Medicine*, **42**, 899–912.

Heatley, R. V., Calcraft, B. J., Rhodes, J., Owen, E., and Evans, B. K. (1975). Disodium cromoglycate in the treatment of chronic proctitis. *Gut*, **16**, 559–63.

Heiner, D. C., Lahey, M. E., Wilson, J. F., Gerrard, J. W., Schwachman, H., and Khaw, K. T. (1962). Precipitins to antigens of wheat and cow's milk in coeliac disease. *Journal of Pediatrics*, **61**, 813–30.

Hemmings, W. A., and Williams, E. W. (1978). Transport of large breakdown products of dietary protein through the gut wall. *Gut*, **19**, 715–23.

Henderson, A., and Hishon, S. (1978). Crohn's disease responding to oral disodium cromoglycate. *Lancet*, **1**, 109–10.

Hendrick, D. J., Faux, J. A., Anand, B., Piris, J., and Marshall, R. (1978). Is the bird fancier's lung associated with coeliac disease? *Thorax*, **33**, 425–8.

Hepner, G. W., Jowsey, J., Arnaud, C., Gordon, S., Black, J., Roginsky, M., Moo, H. F., and Young, J. F. (1978). Osteomalacia and coeliac disease. Response to 25 hydroxy vitamin D. *American Journal of Medicine*, **65**, 1015–20.

Hobbs, J. R., and Hepner, G. W. (1968). Deficiency of γ M in coeliac disease. *Lancet*, **1**, 217–20.

Hodgson, H. J. F., Davies, R. J., Gent, A. E., and Hodson, M. E. (1976). Atopic disorders and adult coeliac disease. *Lancet*, **1**, 115–17.

Hoffbrand, A. V. (1974). Anaemia in adult coeliac disease. *Clinics in Gastroenterology*, **3**, 71–89.

Hollander, D., Muralidhara, K. S., and Zimmerman, A. (1979). Vitamin D3 intestinal absorption in vivo: influence of fatty acids, bile salts and perfusate pH on absorption. *Gut*, **19**, 267–72.

Holmes, G. K. T., Asquith, P., and Cooke, W. T. (1976). Cell mediated immunity to gluten fraction III in adult coeliac disease. *Clinical and Experimental Immunology*, **24**, 259–65.

Holmes, G. K. T., Asquith, P., Stokes, P. L., and Cooke, W. T. (1974). Cellular infiltrate of jejunal biopsies in adult coeliac disease in relation to gluten withdrawal. *Gut*, **15**, 278–83.

Holmes, G. K. T., Stokes, P. L., Sorahan, T. M., Prior, P., Waterhouse, J. A. H., and Cooke, W. T. (1976). Coeliac disease, gluten free diet and malignancy. *Gut*, **17**, 612–19.

Hood, J., and Mason, A. M. S. (1970). Diffuse pulmonary disease with transfer defect occurring with coeliac disease. *Lancet*, **1**, 445–8.

Housley, J., Asquith, P., and Cooke, W. T. (1969). Immune response to gluten in adult coeliac disease. *British Medical Journal*, **2**, 159–61.

Howland, J. (1921). Prolonged intolerance to carbohydrates. *Transactions of the American Pediatric Society*, **33**, 11–19.

Isaacson, P., and Wright, D. H. (1978). Intestinal lymphoma associated with malabsorption. *Lancet*, **1**, 67–70.

Jackson, P. G., Lessof, M. H., Baker, R. W. R., Ferrett, J., and MacDonald, D. M. (1981). Intestinal permeability in patients with eczema and food allergy. *Lancet*, **1**, 1285–6.

James, A. H. (1977). Breakfast and Crohn's disease. *British Medical Journal*, **1**, 943–5.

Jewell, D. P., and Truelove, S. C. (1972). Circulating antibodies to cow's milk proteins in ulcerative colitis. *Gut*, **13**, 796–801.

Jonas, A. (1978). Wheat sensitive — but not coeliac. *Lancet*, **2**, 1047.

Jones, D. B., Kerr, G. D., Parker, J. H., and Wilson, R. S. E. (1981). Dietary allergy and specific IgE in ulcerative colitis. *Journal of the Royal Society of Medicine*, **74**, 292–3.

Kasarda, D. D., Bernadin, J. E., and Qualset, C. O. (1976). Relationship of gliadin protein components to chromosomes in hexaploid wheats (*Triticum aestivum* L). *Proceedings of the National Academy of Sciences of the United States of America*, **73**, 3646.

Katz, S. I., and Strober, W. (1978). The pathogenesis of dermatitis herpetiformis. *Journal of Investigative Dermatology*, **70**, 63–75.

Kazer, H. (1961). Diagnose und klinik der coeliakie. *Annales Paediatrica*, **197**, 320–34.

Kesavan, V., and Noronha, J. M. (1978). An ATPase dependant radiosensitive acidic microclimate essential for intestinal folate absorption. *Journal of Physiology*, **280**, 1–7.

Klein, N. C., Hargrove, R. L., Sleisenger, M. H., and Jeffries, G. H. (1970). Eosinophilic gastroenteritis. *Medicine (Baltimore)*, **49**, 299–319.

Kocoshis, S., and Gryboski, J. D. (1979). Use of cromolyn in combined gastrointestinal allergy. *Journal of the American Medical Association*, **242**, 1169–73.

Kosnai, I., Kuitunen, P., and Siimes, M. A. (1979). Iron deficiency in children with coeliac disease on treatment with gluten free diet. Role of intestinal blood loss. *Archives of Disease in Childhood*, **54**, 375–8.

Krainick, H. G., Debatin, F., Gautier, E., Tobler, R., and Velasco, J. A. (1958). Additional research on the injurious effect of wheat flour in coeliac disease. I. Acute gliadin reaction — gliadin shock. *Helvetica Paediatrica Acta*, **13**, 432–54.

Kuitenen, P., Visakorpi, J. K., Savilahti, E., and Pelkonen, P. (1975). Malabsorption syndrome with cow's milk intolerance. Clinical findings and course in 54 cases. *Archives of Disease in Childhood*, **50**, 351–6.

Lancaster-Smith, M., Kumar, P. J., and Dawson, A. M. (1975). The cellular infiltrate of the jejunum in adult coeliac disease and dermatitis herpetiformis following the reintroduction of dietary gluten. *Gut*, **16**, 683–8.

Lancaster-Smith, M., Kumar, P. J., Marks, R., Clark, M. L., and Dawson, A. M. (1974). Jejunal mucosal immunoglobulin-containing cells and jejunal fluid immunoglobulins in adult coeliac disease and dermatitis herpetiformis. *Gut*, **15**, 371–6.

Lancaster-Smith, M., Packer, S., Kumar, P. J., and Harries, J. T. (1976a). Cellular infiltration of the jejunum after reintroduction of dietary gluten in children with treated coeliac disease. *Journal of Clinical Pathology*, **29**, 587–91.

Lancaster-Smith, M., Packer, S., Kumar, P. J., and Harries, J. T. (1975b). Immunological phenomena in the jejunum and serum after reintroduction of dietary gluten in children with treated coeliac disease. *Journal of Clinical Pathology*, **29**, 592–7.

Lancaster-Smith, M., Perrin, J., Swarbrick, E. T., and Wright, J. T. (1974). Coeliac disease and autoimmunity. *Postgraduate Medical Journal*, **50**, 45–8.

Leeming, R. J., and Blair, J. A. (1980). Serum crithidia levels in disease. *Biochemical Medicine*, **23**, 122–5.

Leeming, R. J., Blair, J. A., Melikian, V., and O'Gorman, D. J. (1976). Biopterin derivatives in human body fluids and tissues. *Journal of Clinical Pathology*, **29**, 444–51.

Leinbach, G. E., and Rubin, C. E. (1970). Eosinophilic gastroenteritis: a simple reaction to food allergens. *Gastroenterology*, **59**, 874–89.

Lloyd, G., Green, F. H. Y., Fox, H., Mani, V., and Turnberg, L. A. (1975). Mast cells and immunoglobulin E in inflammatory bowel disease. *Gut*, **16**, 861–6.

Loeb, P. M., Strober, W., Falchuk, Z. M., and Laster, L. (1971). Incorporation of L-Leucine[14]C into immunoglobulins by jejunal biopsies of patients with coeliac sprue and other gastrointestinal diseases. *Journal of Clinical Investigation*, **50**, 559–69.

Logan, R. F. A., Gillon, J., Ferrington, C., and Ferguson, A. (1981). Reduction of gastrointestinal protein loss by elemental diet in Crohn's disease of the small bowel. *Gut*, **22**, 383–7.

Lucas, M. L., Cooper, B. T., Lei, F. H., Johnson, I. T., Holmes, G. K. T., Blair, J. A., and Cooke, W. T. (1978). Acid microclimate in coeliac and Crohn's disease: a model for folate malabsorption. *Gut*, **19**, 735–42.

MacDonald, T. T., and Ferguson, A. (1976). Hypersensitivity reactions in the small intestine. Effect of allograft rejection on mucosal architecture and lymphoid cell infiltrate. *Gut*, **17**, 81–91.

MacDonald, W. C., Dobbins, W. O., and Rubin, C. E. (1965). Studies of the familial nature of coeliac sprue using biopsy of the small intestine. *New England Journal of Medicine*, **272**, 448-56.

MacLaurin, B. P., Cooke, W. T., and Ling, N. R. (1971). Impaired lymphocyte reactivity against tumour cells in patients with coeliac disease. *Gut*, **12**, 794-800.

Magalhaes, A. F. N., Peters, T. J., and Doe, W. F. (1974). Studies on the nature and significance of connective tissue antibodies in adult coeliac disease and Crohn's disease. *Gut*, **15**, 284-8.

Mallas, E. G., Williamson, N., Cooper, B. T., and Cooke, W. T. (1977). IgA class reticulin antibodies in relatives of patients with coeliac disease. *Gut*, **18**, 647-50.

Mani, V., Lloyd, G., Green, F. H. Y., Fox, H., and Turnberg, L. A. (1976). Treatment of ulcerative colitis with oral disodium cromoglycate. *Lancet*, **1**, 439-41.

Marsh, G. W., and Stewart, J. S. (1970). Splenic function in adult coeliac disease. *British Journal of Haematology*, **19**, 445-57.

Mawhinney, J., and Tomkin, G. H. (1971). Gluten enteropathy associated with selective IgA deficiency. *Lancet*, **2**, 121-4.

McCarthy, C. F., Fraser, I. D., Evans, K. T., and Read, A. E. (1966). Lymphoreticular dysfunction in idiopathic steatorrhoea. *Gut*, **7**, 140-8.

McNeish, A. S., and Anderson, C. M. (1974). The disorder in childhood. *Clinics in Gastroenterology*, **3**, 127-44.

McNicholl, B., Egan-Mitchell, B., and Fottrell, P. F. (1979). Variability of gluten tolerance in treated childhood coeliac disease. *Gut*, **20**, 126-32.

Melvin, K. E. W., Hepner, G. W., Bordier, P., Neale, G., and Joplin, G. F. (1970). Calcium metabolism and bone pathology in adult coeliac disease. *Quarterly Journal of Medicine*, **39**, 83-113.

Misra, R. C., Kasthuri, D., and Chuttani, H. K. (1966). Adult coeliac disease in the tropics. *British Medical Journal*, **2**, 1230-2.

Mohammed, I., Holborow, E. J., Fry, L., Thompson, B. R., Hoffbrand, A. V., and Stewart, J. S. (1976). Multiple immune complexes and hypocomplementaemia in dermatitis herpetiformis and coeliac disease. *Lancet*, **2**, 487-90.

Montgomery, R. D., and Shearer, A. C. I. (1974). The cell population of the upper jejunal mucosa in tropical sprue and post-infective malabsorption. *Gut*, **15**, 387-91.

Moss, A. J., Waterhouse, C., and Terry, R. (1965). Gluten sensitive enteropathy with osteomalacia but without steatorrhoea. *New England Journal of Medicine*, **272**, 825-30.

Mowbray, J. F., Hoffbrand, A. V., Holborow, E. J., Seah, P. P., and Fry, L. (1973). Circulating immune complexes in dermatitis herpetiformis. *Lancet*, **1**, 400-2.

Mylotte, M., Egan-Mitchell, B., McCarthy, C. F., and McNicholl, B. (1973). Coeliac disease in the West of Ireland. *British Medical Journal*, **3**, 498-9.

Nassim, J. R., Saville, P., Cooke, P., and Mulligan, L. (1958). The effects of vitamin D and gluten free diet in idiopathic steatorrhoea. *Quarterly Journal of Medicine*, **28**, 141-62.

O'Donoghue, D. P., Swarbrick, E. T., and Kumar, P. J. (1979). Type I hypersensitivity reactions in coeliac disease. *Gastroenterology*, **76**, 1211.

Padykula, H. A., Strauss, E. W., Ladman, A. J., and Gardner, F. H. (1961). A morphologic and histochemical analysis of the human jejunal epithelium in non-tropical sprue. *Gastroenterology*, **40**, 735-65.

Parsons, L. G. (1932). Coeliac disease. *American Journal of Diseases of Children*, **43**, 1293-1346.

Paulley, J. W. (1954). Observations on the aetiology of idiopathic steatorrhoea, jejunal and lymph node biopsies. *British Medical Journal*, **2**, 1318-21.

Paulley, J. W. (1959). Emotion and personality aetiology of steatorrhoea. *American Journal of Digestive Disease*, 4, 352–60.

Pena, A. S., Mann, D. L., Hague, N. E., Heck, J. A., Van Leeuwen, A., and Van Rood, J. J. (1978). Genetic basis of gluten sensitive enteropathy. *Gastroenterology*, 75, 230–5.

Pena, A. S., and Truelove, S. C. (1973). Hypolactasia and ulcerative colitis. *Gastroenterology*, 64, 400–4.

Phelan, J. J., Stevens, F. M., McNicholl, B., Fottrell, P. F., and McCarthy, C. F. (1977). Coeliac disease: the abolition of gliadin toxicity by enzymes from *Aspergillus niger*. *Clinical Science and Molecular Medicine*, 53, 35–43.

Pock-Steen, O. C. (1973). The role of gluten, milk and other dietary proteins in chronic or intermittent dyspepsia. *Clinical Allergy*, 3, 373–83.

Poynton, F. J., Armstrong, R. R., and Nabarro, D. N. (1914). A contribution to the study of a group of cases of chronic recurrent diarrhoea in childhood. *British Journal of Childhood Diseases*, 11, 145–55, 193–201.

Rawcliffe, P. M., and Truelove, S. C. (1978). Breakfast and Crohn's disease — I. *British Medical Journal*, 3, 539–40.

Reunala, T., Blomqvist, K., Tarpila, S., Halme, H., and Kangas, K. (1977). Gluten-free diet in dermatitis herpetiformis. I. Clinical response of skin lesions in 81 patients. *British Journal of Dermatology*, 97, 473–80.

Rudman, D., Galambos, J. T., Wenger, J., and Achord, J. L. (1971). Adverse effects of dietary gluten in four patients with regional enteritis. *American Journal of Clinical Nutrition*, 24, 1068–73.

Schedl, H. P., and Clifton, J. A. (1963). Solute and water absorption by the human small intestine. *Nature*, 199, 1264–7.

Scott, B. B., and Losowsky, M. S. (1975). Coeliac disease. A cause of various associated diseases? *Lancet*, 2, 956–7.

Scott, B. B., and Losowsky, M. S. (1976). Cell mediated autoimmunity in coeliac disease. *Clinical and Experimental Immunology*, 26, 243–6.

Seah, P. P., Fry, L., Mazaheri, M. R., Mowbray, J. F., Hoffbrand, A. V., and Holborow, E. J. (1973). Alternate pathway complement fixation by IgA in the skin in dermatitis herpetiformis. *Lancet*, 2, 175–7.

Sencer, W. (1957). Neurologic manifestations in the malabsorption syndrome. *Journal of the Mount Sinai Hospital*, 24, 331–45.

Sewell, P., Cooke, W. T., Cox, E. V., and Meynell, M. J. (1963). Milk intolerance in gastrointestinal disorders. *Lancet*, 2, 1132–5.

Sharpe, G. W. G., and Hynie, S. (1971). Stimulation of intestinal adenycyclase by cholera toxin. *Nature*, 229, 266–9.

Sheldon, W. (1949). Coeliac disease: a relation between dietary starch and fat absorption. *Archives of Disease in Childhood*, 24, 81–7.

Sheldon, W. (1959). Coeliac disease. *Pediatrics*, 23, 132–45.

Shenoi, P. M., Smits, B. J., and Davidson, S. (1966). Massive removal of small bowel during criminal abortion. *British Medical Journal*, 2, 929–31.

Shiner, M., and Ballard, J. (1972). Antigen–antibody reactions in jejunal mucosa in childhood coeliac disease after gluten challenge. *Lancet*, 1, 1202–5.

Shiner, R. J., and Ballard, J. (1973). Mucosal secretory IgA and secretory piece in adult coeliac disease. *Gut*, 14, 778–83.

Sikora, K., Anand, B. S., Truelove, S. C., Ciclitira, P. J., and Offord, R. E. (1976). Stimulation of lymphocytes from patients with coeliac disease by a subfraction of gluten. *Lancet*, 2, 389–91.

Silkoff, K., Hallak, A., Yegena, L., Rozen, P., Mayberry, J. F., Rhodes, J., and

Newcombe, R. G. (1980). Consumption of refined carbohydrate by patients with Crohn's disease in Tel-Aviv-Yato. *Postgraduate Medical Journal*, **56**, 842–6.

Smith, I., Clayton, B. E., and Wolff, O. H. (1975). New variant of phenylketonuria with progressive neurological illness unresponsive to phenylalanine restriction. *Lancet*, **1**, 1108–11.

Sterchi, E. E., and Woodley, J. F. (1978). Peptides of the human intestinal brush border membrane. In: *Perspectives in Coeliac Disease* (eds B. McNicholl, C. F. McCarthy, and F. P. Fottrell). MTP Press, Lancaster, pp.437–49.

Stevens, F. M., Lloyd, R. S., Geraghty, S. M. J., Reynolds, M. T. G., Sarsfield, M. J., McNicholl, B., Fottrell, P. F., Wright, R., and McCarthy, C. F. (1977). Schizophrenia and coeliac disease—the nature of the relationship. *British Journal of Psychological Medicine*, **7**, 259–63.

Still, G. F. (1918). Coeliac disease. *Lancet*, **2**, 163–6, 193–7, 227–9.

Stokes, P. L., Asquith, P., Holmes, G. K. T., Mackintosh, P., and Cooke, W. T. (1972). Histocompatibility antigens associated with adult coeliac disease. *Lancet*, **2**, 162–4.

Stokes, P. L., Ferguson, R., Holmes, G. K. T., and Cooke, W. T. (1976). Familial aspects of coeliac disease. *Quarterly Journal of Medicine*, **45**, 567–82.

Stokes, P. L., Holmes, G. K. T., and Smits, B. J. (1972). Immunoglobulin levels in families with coeliac disease. *Lancet*, **2**, 608.

Swinson, C. M., and Levi, A. J. (1980). Is coeliac disease underdiagnosed? *British Medical Journal*, **281**, 1258–60.

Taylor, K. B., Thompson, D. L., Truelove, S. C., and Wright, R. (1961). An immunological study of coeliac disease and idiopathic steatorrhoea. *British Medical Journal*, **2**, 1727–31.

Taylor, K. B., and Truelove, S. C. (1961). Circulating antibodies to milk proteins in ulcerative colitis. *British Medical Journal*, **2**, 924–9.

Teisberg, P., Fausa, O., Baklien, K., and Akesson, I. (1977). Complement system studies in adult coeliac disease. *Scandinavian Journal of Gastroenterology*, **12**, 873–6.

Thornton, J. R., Emmett, P. M., and Heaton, K. W. (1979). Diet and Crohn's disease: characteristics of the pre-illness diet. *British Medical Journal*, **2**, 762–4.

Townley, R. R., and Anderson, C. M. (1967). Coeliac disease. A review. *Ergebnisse der Inneren Medizin und Kinderheilkunde*, **26**, 1–44.

Trewby, P. N., Chipping, P. M., Palmer, S. J., Roberts, P. D., Lewis, S. M., and Stewart, J. S. (1981). Splenic atrophy in adult coeliac disease: is it reversible? *Gut*, **22**, 628–32.

Truelove, S. C. (1961). Ulcerative colitis provoked by milk. *British Medical Journal*, **1**, 154–60.

Van de Kamer, J. H., Weijers, H. A., and Dicke, W. K. (1953). Coeliac disease. IV. An investigation into the injurious constituents of wheat in connection with their action on patients with coeliac disease. *Acta Paediatrica Scandinavica*, **42**, 223–31.

Visakorpi, J. K. (1979). Milk allergy and the gastrointestinal tract in children. In: *Immunology of the Gastrointestinal Tract* (ed. P. Asquith). Churchill-Livingstone, Edinburgh, pp.183–94.

Volpe, R. (1977). The role of autoimmunity in hypoendocrine and hyperendocrine function. *Annals of Internal Medicine*, **87**, 86–99.

Walia, B. N. S., Sidhu, J. K., Tandon, B. N., Ghai, O. P., and Bhargava, S. (1966). Coeliac disease in North Indian children. *British Medical Journal*, **2**, 1233–4.

Wall, A. J., Douglas, A. P., Booth, C. C., and Pearse, A. G. E. (1970). Response of the jejunal mucosa in adult coeliac disease to oral prednisolone. *Gut*, **11**, 7–14.

Wattenberg, L. W. (1966). Carcinogenic-detoxifying mechanisms in the gastrointestinal tract. *Gastroenterology*, **51**, 932–5.

Weinstein, W. M. (1974). Latent coeliac sprue. *Gastroenterology*, **66**, 489–93.

Weir, D. G., Brown, J. P., Freedman, D. S., and Scott, J. M. (1973). The absorption of the disastereoisomers of 5-methyltetrahydropteroylglutamate in man: a carrier-mediated process. *Clinical Science and Molecular Medicine*, **45**, 625–31.

Weiser, M. M., and Douglas, A. P. (1976). An alternative mechanism for gluten toxicity in coeliac disease. *Lancet*, **1**, 567–9.

Weiser, M. M., and Douglas, A. P. (1978). Cell surface glycosyltransferases of the enterocyte in coeliac disease. In: *Perspectives in Coeliac Disease* (eds B. McNicholl, C. F. McCarthy, and P. F. Fottrell). MTP Press, Lancaster, pp.451–8.

Williamson, N., Asquith, P., Stokes, P. L., Jowett, A. W., and Cooke, W. T. (1976). Anticonnective tissue and other antitissue 'antibodies' in the sera of patients with coeliac disease compared with findings in a mixed hospital population. *Journal of Clinical Pathology*, **29**, 484–94.

Wraith, D. G., Merrett, J., Roth, A., Yman, L., and Merrett, T. G. (1979). Recognition of food-allergic patients and their allergens by the RAST technique and clinical investigation. *Clinical Allergy*, **9**, 25–36.

Wray, D. (1981). Gluten-sensitive recurrent aphthous stomatitis. *Digestive Diseases and Sciences*, **26**, 737–40.

Wright, R., and Truelove, S. C. (1965a). A controlled therapeutic trial of various diets in ulcerative colitis. *British Medical Journal*, **2**, 138–41.

Wright, R., and Truelove, S. C. (1965b). Circulating antibodies to dietary proteins in ulcerative colitis. *British Medical Journal*, **2**, 142–4.

Wright, R., and Truelove, S. C. (1966). Circulating and tissue eosinophils in ulcerative colitis. *American Journal of Digestive Disease*, **11**, 831–46.

Zioudrou, C., Streaty, R. A., and Klee, W. A. (1979). Opioid peptides derived from food proteins. The exorphins. *Journal of Biological Chemistry*, **254**, 2446–9.

Index